# Psychiatric–Legal Decision Making by the Mental Health Practitioner

# An Einstein Psychiatry Publication

Publication Series of the Department of Psychiatry
Albert Einstein College of Medicine of Yeshiva University
New York, NY

*Editor-in-Chief*     Herman M. van Praag, M.D., Ph.D.
*Associate Editor*     Demitri Papolos, M.D.

### Editorial Board

1. CONTEMPORARY APPROACHES TO PSYCHOLOGICAL ASSESSMENT
*Edited by Scott Wetzler, Ph.D. & Martin M. Katz, Ph.D.*

2. COMPUTER APPLICATIONS IN PSYCHIATRY AND PSYCHOLOGY
*Edited by David Baskin, Ph.D.*

3. VIOLENCE AND SUICIDALITY: PERSPECTIVES IN CLINICAL
AND PSYCHOBIOLOGICAL RESEARCH
*Edited by Herman M. van Praag, M.D., Ph.D.*
*Robert Plutchik, Ph.D., & Alan Apter, M.D.*

4. THE ROLE OF SEROTONIN IN PSYCHIATRIC DISORDERS
*Edited by Serena-Lynn Brown, M.D., Ph.D*
*& Herman M. van Praag, M.D., Ph.D.*

5. POSITIVE AND NEGATIVE SYNDROMES IN SCHIZOPHRENIA:
ASSESSMENT AND RESEARCH
*by Stanley R. Kay, Ph.D.*

6. NEW BIOLOGICAL VISTAS ON SCHIZOPHRENIA
*Edited by Jean-Pierre Lindenmayer, M.D.*
*& Stanley R. Kay, Ph.D.*

7. "MAKE-BELIEVES" IN PSYCHIATRY, OR THE PERILS OF PROGRESS
*by Herman M. van Praag, M.D., Ph.D.*

8. GENETIC STUDIES IN AFFECTIVE DISORDERS: BASIC METHODS,
CURRENT DIRECTIONS, AND CRITICAL RESEARCH ISSUES
*Edited by Demitri F. Papolos, M.D.*
*& Herbert M. Lachman, M.D.*

9. PSYCHIATRIC–LEGAL DECISION MAKING BY THE MENTAL HEALTH PRACTITIONER:
THE CLINICIAN AS DE FACTO MAGISTRATE
*Edited by Harvey Bluestone, M.D.,*
*Sheldon Travin, M.D., & Douglas B. Marlowe, J.D., Ph.D.*

*Einstein Psychiatry Publication No. 9*

# Psychiatric–Legal Decision Making by the Mental Health Practitioner

## The Clinician as de facto Magistrate

---

*Edited by*

*HARVEY BLUESTONE*

*SHELDON TRAVIN*

*DOUGLAS B. MARLOWE*

A Wiley-Interscience Publication

John Wiley & Sons, Inc.

New York • Chichester • Brisbane • Toronto • Singapore

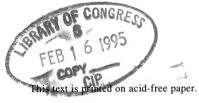

This publication is designed to provide accurate and
authoritative information in regard to the subject
matter covered. It is sold with the understanding that
the publisher is not engaged in rendering legal, accounting,
or other professional services. If legal advice or other
expert assistance is required, the services of a competent
professional person should be sought. *From a Declaration
of Principles jointly adopted by a Committee of the
American Bar Association and a Committee of Publishers.*

*Library of Congress Cataloging in Publication Data:*

Psychiatric–legal decision making by the mental health practitioner :
    the clinician as de facto magistrate / edited by Harvey Bluestone,
    Sheldon Travin, Douglas B. Marlowe.
        p.    cm. — (Publication series of the Department of Psychiatry
    Albert Einstein College of Medicine of Yeshiva University : 9)
        Includes index.
        ISBN 0-471-00431-6 (cloth : alk. paper)
        1. Psychiatry—Decision making.   2. Forensic psychiatry—Decision
    Making.   4. Ethics, Medical.   W 740 P9725 1994]
    RC455.2.D42P785    1994
    614'.1—dc20
    DNLM/DLC
                                                                93-5998

Printed in the United States of America

10 9 8 7 6 5 4 3 2 1

# Contributors

**Karen Blank, M.D.** Assistant Clinical Professor of Psychiatry, University of Connecticut School of Medicine, Farmington, Connecticut.

**Harvey Bluestone, M.D.** Professor of Psychiatry, Albert Einstein College of Medicine; Director, Department of Psychiatry, Bronx-Lebanon Hospital Center, Bronx, New York.

**Linda T. Cahill, M.D.** Assistant Professor of Pediatrics, Albert Einstein College of Medicine; Director, Child Protective Services Program, North Central Bronx Hospital; Director, Child Protection Center, Montefiore Medical Center, Bronx, New York.

**Christina Casals-Ariet, M.D., J.D.** Assistant Professor of Psychiatry, Albert Einstein College of Medicine; Bronx-Lebanon Hospital Center, Bronx, New York.

**Thomas Garrick, M.D.** Associate Professor of Psychiatry, University of California at Los Angeles; Chief, General Hospital Psychiatry, West Los Angeles Veterans Administration Medical Center, Los Angeles, California.

**Elisabeth N. Gibbings, Psy.D.** Director of Outpatient Services and The Children's Center, HCA Rockford Center, Newark, Delaware.

**Lynn D. Hamberg, M.Ed., CSW.** Social Worker, Child Protection Center, Montefiore Medical Center, Bronx, New York.

**Leah E. Harrison, MSN, CPNP.** Assistant Director, Child Protection Center, Montefiore Medical Center, Bronx, New York.

**Hyung Kon Lee, M.D.** Associate Professor of Psychiatry, Albert Einstein College of Medicine; Director of Substance Abuse Treatment Services, Bronx-Lebanon Hospital Center, Bronx, New York.

v

**Ruth Macklin, Ph.D.** Professor of Bioethics, Department of Epidemiology and Social Medicine, Albert Einstein College of Medicine, Bronx, New York.

**Douglas B. Marlowe, J.D., Ph.D.** Research Assistant Professor and Clinical Supervisor, Division of Addiction Research and Treatment, Hahnemann University, Camden, New Jersey and Philadelphia, Pennsylvania.

**Carol R. Perlman, CSW.** Social Worker, Harriet Feinman Child Protection Project, Child Protection Center, Montefiore Medical Center, Bronx, New York.

**Stephen Rachlin, M.D.** Chairman, Department of Psychiatry and Psychology, Nassau County Medical Center, East Meadow, New York; Professor of Clinical Psychiatry, State University of New York, Stony Brook.

**Richard Rosner, M.D.** Associate Commissioner for Forensic Mental Health Services and Medical Director, Forensic Psychiatry Clinic, New York City Department of Mental Health, Mental Retardation and Alcoholism Services; Clinical Professor of Psychiatry, New York University School of Medicine, New York, New York.

**Robert L. Sadoff, M.D.** Clinical Professor of Psychiatry and Director of the Center for Studies in Social-Legal Psychiatry, University of Pennsylvania, Philadelphia, Pennsylvania.

**Julie B. Sadoff, M.A., J.D.** Master of Arts in Philosophy; Member of the Bar, Commonwealth of Pennsylvania.

**Jose Arturo Sanchez-Lacay, M.D.** Assistant Professor of Psychiatry, Albert Einstein College of Medicine; Bronx-Lebanon Hospital Center, Bronx, New York.

**Harold I. Schwartz, M.D.** Director, Department of Psychiatry, Hartford General Hospital, Hartford, Connecticut.

**Allan M. Tepper, J.D., Psy.D.** Private Practice, Philadelphia, Pennsylvania.

**Sheldon Travin, M.D.** Professor of Psychiatry, Albert Einstein College of Medicine; Associate Director, Department of Psychiatry, Bronx-Lebanon Hospital Center, Bronx, New York.

**Gopalakrishna Upadhya, M.D.** Assistant Professor of Psychiatry, Albert Einstein College of Medicine; Chief, Consultation/Liaison Department, Bronx-Lebanon Hospital Center, Bronx, New York.

**Ricardo M. Vela, M.D.** Assistant Professor of Psychiatry, Albert Einstein College of Medicine; Child and Adolescent Services, Bronx-Lebanon Hospital Center, Bronx, New York.

**Robert Weinstock, M.D.** Associate Clinical Professor of Psychiatry, University of California at Los Angeles; Co-Director, Forensic Psychiatry Fellowship Program, University of California at Los Angeles; Director, Out-Patient Psychiatric Consultation, West Los Angeles Veterans Administration Medical Center, Los Angeles, California.

# A Note on the Series

Psychiatry is in a state of flux. The excitement springs in part from internal changes, such as the development and official acceptance (at least in the U.S.A.) of an operationalized, multiaxial classification system of behavioral disorders (the DSM-III), the increasing sophistication of methods to measure abnormal human behavior and the impressive expansion of biological and psychological treatment modalities. Exciting developments are also taking place in fields relating to psychiatry; in molecular (brain) biology, genetics, brain imaging, drug development, epidemiology, experimental psychology, to mention only a few striking examples.

More generally speaking, psychiatry is moving, still relatively slowly, but irresistibly, from a more philosophical, contemplative orientation, to that of an empirical science. From the fifties on, biological psychiatry has been a major catalyst of that process. It provided the mother discipline with a third cornerstone, that is, neurobiology, the other two being psychology and medical sociology. In addition, it forced the profession into the direction of standardization of diagnoses and of assessment of abnormal behavior. Biological psychiatry provided psychiatry not only with a new basic science and with new treatment modalities, but also with the tools, the methodology and the mentality to operate within the confines of an empirical science, the only framework in which a medical discipline can survive.

In other fields of psychiatry, too, one discerns a gradual trend towards scientification. Psychological treatment techniques are standardized and manuals developed to make these skills more easily transferable. Methods registering treatment outcome—traditionally used in the behavioral/cognitive field—are now more and more requested and, hence, developed for dynamic forms of psychotherapy as well. Social and community psychiatry, until the sixties more firmly rooted in humanitarian ideals and social awareness than in empirical studies, profited greatly from its liaison with the social sciences and the expansion of psychiatric epidemiology.

Let there be no misunderstanding. Empiricism does *not imply* that it is only the measurable that counts. Psychiatry would be mutilated if it would neglect that which cannot be captured by numbers. It *does imply* that what is measurable should be measured. Progress in psychiatry is dependent on ideas and on experiment. Their linkage is inseparable.

This Series, published under the auspices of the Department of Psychiatry of the Albert Einstein College of Medicine, Montefiore Medical Center, is meant to keep track of important developments in our profession, to summarize what has been achieved in particular fields, and to bring together the viewpoints obtained from disparate vantage points—in short, to capture some of the ongoing excitement in modern psychiatry, both in its clinical and experimental dimensions. The Department of Psychiatry at Albert Einstein College of Medicine hosts the Series, but naturally welcomes contributions from others.

Bernie Mazel originally generated the idea—an ambitious plan which we all felt was worthy of pursuit. The edifice of psychiatry is impressive, but still somewhat flawed in its foundations. May this Series contribute to consolidation of its infrastructure.

HERMAN M. VAN PRAAG, M.D., PH.D.
*Professor and Chairman*
*Academic Psychiatric Center*
*University of Limburg*
*Maastricht*
*The Netherlands*

# *Preface*

This book makes a significant contribution to the monograph series published under the auspices of the Department of Psychiatry of the Albert Einstein College of Medicine/Montefiore Medical Center. Its principal focus is to assist clinicians in a crucial area of psychiatric practice, namely making vital decisions on treatment and dispositional issues which have profound legal and ethical implications. Clinical care has changed significantly in recent years. Increasingly, mental health clinicians have had to contend with myriad legal and ethical concerns regarding the provision of psychiatric treatment for their patients.

The major theme of the book as manifested in the title, *Psychiatric–Legal Decision Making by the Mental Health Practitioner: The Clinician as de facto Magistrate* is that psychiatric decisions having legal and ethical implications are made by practitioners in clinical settings rather than in formal legal arenas. Because clinicians are making these decisions it is important that they acquire knowledge of and familiarity with the decision-making process. This book provides substantial help to clinicians in this area. Especially helpful are case examples and discussions by experienced professionals on important clinical dilemmas. These dilemmas are faced by practitioners on a routine basis.

With its emphasis on practicality and usefulness for clinicians with their day-to-day problems, the book fills a substantial niche in the publication series.

HARVEY BLUESTONE
SHELDON TRAVIN
DOUGLAS B. MARLOWE

xi

# Contents

# Introduction

This book is designed to help clinicians make essential psychiatric–legal decisions in their work in general hospitals. Such decisions involve the question of when, or whether, to take therapeutic actions regarding patients in view of the statutes, regulations, and judicial rulings in various jurisdictions. Clinicians are, in fact, making such decisions, many of which have profound legal and ethical implications, without sufficient background in these areas. The principal purposes of this book are to make clinicians aware of the legal and ethical aspects of their day-to-day practice and to present relevant background material on these matters so that they can make better-informed decisions.

The clinical activities of professionals in the general hospital often encompass aspects of legal decision making. Although, in a strict sense of the term, such decision making is a judicial prerogative, in the hospital setting comparatively few of these decisions are ever made by a judge. The clinician is indeed the one who makes decisions on a wide range of psychiatric–legal issues, thereby functioning as a de facto decision maker—although the vast majority of these clinicians are not forensic specialists, nor are they specifically trained in legal matters. But clinicians do gain some familiarity with the legal implications of their work through clinical experience, and this book attempts to complement and expand on that knowledge. Acquiring knowledge about and sensitivity to these issues is crucial because of the increasing impingement of the law on psychiatric practice in recent years. Therefore, this work should enable practitioners to function more confidently and effectively.

The book's focus on psychiatric–legal decision making in general hospitals reflects not only the professional experiences of the editors, but also the increasingly prominent position assumed by the general hospital in the provision of psychiatric care in the United States, primarily by virtue of its easy accessibility and expanding range of services. Indeed, the majority of patients with psychiatric disorders are now being admitted to short-term general hospitals rather than to psychiatric hospitals. Consequently, clinicians treat a large number of psychiatric disorders, including psychoses, substance abuse, and organic brain syndromes—and, in doing so, they have to contend with the multitude of legal regulations and ethical considerations involved in their patients' care.

## OUTLINE OF BOOK

The book is divided into four major groups—Basic Principles, Psychiatric Emergency and Inpatient Services, Outpatient Services, and Special Categories—each of which is subdivided by treatment location or specialized areas. The authors of the various chapters focus on the more prominent legal issues presented in these settings. Of paramount importance in psychiatric emergency services, for example, are such issues as rapid assessment, emergency intervention, and civil commitment. By contrast, on the inpatient service, where there are fewer exigencies justifying emergency treatment, such issues as the right to refuse treatment, consent to special treatment procedures, and participation in research assume greater importance. Other treatment contexts, such as the consultation–liaison service, confront the clinician with issues of competency to give informed consent and "Do Not Resuscitate" orders and to make right-to-die decisions. Rather than organizing this work around underlying legal principles such as privacy, liberty, and competency, the editors instead organized it around treatment contexts so as to make it more accessible to clinicians.

## BASIC PRINCIPLES

Part I on basic principles underscores the importance of both legal and ethical issues that clinicians must consider in clinical decision making. In Chapter 1, Douglas Marlowe, an attorney and psychologist, develops the thesis that clinical decisions, which often encompass legal aspects, are usually made independently of the judicial process. This thesis, supported by case decisions and illustrated by clinical vignettes, portrays the clinician as functioning as a kind of de facto magistrate—hence the title of the chapter, "The de facto Magistrate: Psycholegal Decision Making in Clinical Practice." The psycholegal formulations described serve as a preview for more detailed discussions in the subsequent chapters.

Chapter 2 in this part, "Ethics and Decision Making in Psychiatric Practice in General Hospitals," was written by Ruth Macklin, a professor of bioethics at Albert Einstein College of Medicine and an internationally renowned medical bioethicist. She describes the basic principles of biomedical ethics that were raised in hospital cases presented at rounds, conferences, and seminars in which she participated as a discussant. Macklin emphasizes that ethical principles are frequently in conflict with one another, and explains that the impossibility of simultaneously adhering to conflicting ethical principles gives rise to ethical dilemmas in clinical decision making. An example of an ethical dilemma is that arising from the conflict between the principles of respect for autonomy and beneficence. It should be pointed out that ethical concerns pervade the content of this volume and incorporate many of the principles that Macklin outlines.

## PSYCHIATRIC EMERGENCY AND INPATIENT SERVICES

The chapter on psychiatric emergency services and those on inpatient services are combined into Part II because the majority of involuntary admissions to psychiatric units occur through the emergency room, and because both services are concerned with the need to stabilize the patient immediately or to provide short-term psychiatric care. In addition, a chapter on consultations performed on the general medical wards is included in this section. Chapter 3, "Emergency Room Psychiatric Care in the General Hospital: Major Psychiatric–Legal Considerations," was written by Sheldon Travin, a forensic psychiatrist with considerable experience in an inner-city psychiatric emergency service. He describes the major legal issues relevant to clinical decision making in the assessment and management of patients seen in the emergency room, where an increasing number of persons with multiple psychiatric disorders are being seen. Because of the complex nature of these presentations, the uncertainty of the diagnoses, and the need for rapid decision making, clinicians need to be aware of the legal and ethical issues inherent in working in this setting.

Chapter 4, contributed by Stephen Rachlin, a forensic psychiatrist and chairman of the Department of Psychiatry and Psychology at Nassau County Medical Center, is titled, "Retention and Treatment Issues on the Psychiatric Inpatient Unit." Rachlin describes the recent developments in the law pertaining to involuntary psychiatric hospitalization, which includes both emergency admission and longer-term retention. He also discusses treatment issues, particularly the right to refuse treatment. In Chapter 5, Sheldon Travin, drawing on his experience as Associate Director of Psychiatry at the Bronx-Lebanon Hospital Center, writes about the problem of assaultive patients on the inpatient psychiatric service. In this chapter, "Management of Assaultive Patients on the Psychiatric Unit of the General Hospital: Legal and Ethical Considerations," Travin points out that the problem of violence on psychiatric wards appears to have worsened, and that the legal regulations governing the management of violent patients have become more complex.

Karen Blank, a psychiatrist with experience as a unit chief on an inpatient geriatric psychiatric service, and Harold Schwartz, a forensic psychiatrist and Director of Psychiatry at Hartford General Hospital, have contributed Chapter 6 on "Inpatient Geriatric Psychiatry: Special Legal and Ethical Considerations." The authors present a detailed review of the legal and ethical issues surrounding such topics as informed consent and treatment decisions, confidentiality, electroconvulsive therapy, discharge planning, and elder abuse.

Chapter 7, the last in Part II, coauthored by Robert Weinstock, a forensic psychiatrist and Director of Outpatient Psychiatry Consultation at a Veterans Administration Medical Center (VAMC), and Thomas Garrick, chief of General Hospital Psychiatry at a VAMC, is titled "Consultation–Liaison Psychiatry on the General Medical Wards." Among the topics addressed are tests for determining competency to give informed consent or to refuse consent, issues involved in assessing a patient's capacity to refuse life-sustaining treatment, and concerns about confidentiality and the sharing of information with the referring physician.

## OUTPATIENT SERVICES

Part III on outpatient services reflects the growing diversity of services being offered in some general hospitals. The first contribution in Part III, Chapter 8, "Forensic Problems Encountered in the Practice of Child and Adolescent Psychiatry," was written by Ricardo Vela and José Sanchez-Lacay, both of whom are child–adolescent psychiatrists, and Harvey Bluestone, a forensic psychiatrist and Director of Psychiatry at Bronx-Lebanon Hospital Center. The authors point out that whether or not clinicians like it, they inevitably will be confronted with legal and ethical problems in their day-to-day professional activities. While Vela and Sanchez-Lacay draw upon their daily clinical experiences to recount illustrative case histories, Bluestone, an authority on forensic issues, casts these cases in the framework of the relevant ethical and legal issues.

Chapter 9, "Ethical and Forensic Considerations in Substance Abuse Treatment" by Hyung Kon Lee, chief of the Substance Abuse Services at Bronx-Lebanon Hospital Center, and Harvey Bluestone, underscores the special legal and ethical considerations of confidentiality in substance abuse treatment, of coercive treatment in driving-while-intoxicated (DWI) treatment programs, and of physicians who are impaired as a result of alcoholism or drug dependence. Lee's discussion of cases culled from his vast experience in the field is complemented by Bluestone's further discussion of the relevant forensic issues.

In the final chapter in Part III, Chapter 10, "Partial Hospitalization and Intensive Outpatient Management in the General Hospital: A Unique Clinicolegal Status," Douglas Marlowe and Allan Tepper, both of whom are psychologists and attorneys, and Elisabeth Gibbings, Director of Outpatient Services and Partial Hospitalization Programs at the HCA Rockford Center, describe the common legal, ethical, and administrative issues that need to be confronted in developing innovative partial hospitalization and intensive outpatient case management programs in general hospitals. Among these concerns are the location of the program, specialized programming and treatment planning, patient-selection criteria, regulation of the milieu, setting the ground rules of treatment, and techniques of confrontation and premature disclosure.

## SPECIAL CATEGORIES

The first contributors to Part IV are Gopalakrishna Upadhya, chief of the Consultation–Liaison Service at Bronx-Lebanon Hospital Center, and Harvey Bluestone, whose Chapter 11 is titled "AIDS and Psychiatry in the General Hospital: Legal and Ethical Dilemmas." The authors describe some of the dilemmas that confront clinicians in treating AIDS patients in the general hospital, including the difficulties of managing hospitalized aggressive seropositive patients, many of whom have had lifelong personality disorders. One of the most difficult dilemmas that clinicians face in treating AIDS patients is related to issues of confidentiality, given the legal and ethical concerns about reporting the condition to state authorities and to potential victims of infection.

Chapter 12, "Psychiatric Training, Supervision, and Shared Responsibility: Some Forensic Concerns," is by Richard Rosner, a forensic psychiatrist and past president of the American Academy of Psychiatry and the Law (AAPL). Rosner discusses the phenomenon of shared responsibilities among supervisors and supervisees, and offers general guidelines for a working professional relationship among them in their joint care of the patient. Robert Sadoff, a forensic psychiatrist and a past president of AAPL, and Julie Sadoff, an attorney, coauthored Chapter 13, "The Impaired Health Professional: Legal and Ethical Issues." They review issues relating to the nature of impairment, reporting of the impaired professional, disciplining and treating the professional, and general philosophical and ethical concerns in this area.

Chapter 14, "Child Abuse Reporting in the General Hospital," was written by Linda Cahill, a pediatrician and Director of the Child Protection Center at Montefiore Medical Center; Leah Harrison, a pediatric nurse practitioner and Assistant Director of the Child Protection Center; and Lynn Hamberg and Carol Perlman, social workers in the Child Protection Center. The authors highlight the dramatic increase in the reporting of child abuse and neglect in recent years in the United States. They provide a definition of child "abuse" and "neglect," describe modern child abuse legislation, point out indicators of risk of abuse and neglect, detail techniques of evaluating abuse, and emphasize the increasing concerns about fetal abuse.

Finally, in Chapter 15, "Legal and Ethical Issues in Psychiatric Research," Christina Casals-Ariet, a forensic psychiatrist and attorney, describes the legal and ethical issues that must be addressed in order to conduct research in a hospital setting. She explores the issues of informed consent, competency, institutional review boards (IRBs), and coercion as essential considerations in the protection of vulnerable research subjects.

## DUPLICATION OF SUBJECTS

Although efforts have been made to prevent duplication of material in the various chapters, a certain amount of overlap was unavoidable. This overlap, however, provides somewhat differing perspectives on the same subject, and thus enriches the discussion. As an example, the subject of AIDS is discussed by Macklin in Chapter 2, illustrating the dilemma arising from competing ethical principles, which is further complicated by relevant laws and regulations; by Lee and Bluestone (Chapter 9) in the context of confidentiality issues in substance abuse treatment; and by Upadhya and Bluestone (Chapter 11) with regard to the health-care provider's complicated and often conflicting roles of maintaining the therapeutic relationship, guarding client confidentiality, and protecting the general public.

Another example of the duplication of subject matter is alcoholism. Travin (Chapter 3) presents the case of an acutely intoxicated individual who presents in the emergency room, Lee and Bluestone (Chapter 9) discuss the legal and ethical issues involved in requiring treatment in a driving-while-intoxicated program, and Sadoff and Sadoff (Chapter 13) address alcoholism as an example of physician impairment. Violent behavior and other forms of emergencies are subjects that are described in the chapters on emergency rooms, psychiatric units, and other areas of the hospital. Such duplication is inevitable given the subjects treated in this work. But in addition to enriching the discussion, as pointed out, this duplication reflects a completeness that enables each chapter to stand on its own, and thus makes this book particularly useful to clinicians working in these areas.

## FAMILIARITY WITH LOCAL LAWS

Clinicians should understand that this work is not intended to be formal "legal advice." As indicated earlier, psychiatric–legal decisions are performed in the context of statutes, regulations, and judicial rulings in various jurisdictions. Laws and professional standards are constantly evolving, and the legal mandates may vary from jurisdiction to jurisdiction. The book emphasizes general legal and ethical principles that underlie specific decisions, but reminds the reader that, in addition to knowing these general principles, clinicians also must be familiar with the laws and regulations in their own jurisdictions.

## SUMMARY

This book posits that clinical decisions must be informed by legal and ethical considerations. The contents, as the above overview illustrates, will assist clinicians in their effort to provide psychiatric care that combines clinical expertise with a sensitivity to and respect for the rights of patients as individuals.

HARVEY BLUESTONE
SHELDON TRAVIN
DOUGLAS B. MARLOWE

# PART I
# Basic Principles

# 1

# The de facto Magistrate
## Psycholegal Decision Making in Clinical Practice

DOUGLAS B. MARLOWE

### DEFERENCE TO DECISION-MAKING PRACTICES
### OF HEALTH-CARE PROFESSIONALS

In recent years, health professionals have been expressing increasing
concern about the legal regulation of clinical practice. The sources of
this regulation are so diverse, and the mandates so complex and seemingly contradictory, that it is difficult to understand and reconcile the
existing requirements (Miller, 1986). Significantly, such regulation
brings with it the potential for increased exposure to civil and criminal
liability (Bennett, Bryant, VandenBos, & Greenwood, 1990), and may
interfere with the professional–patient relationship and the process of
clinical decision making (Everstine & Everstine, 1986).

Proponents of increased regulation, however, point out that a lack of
oversight in the past led to extreme abuses, suggesting that health-care
professionals are incapable of developing or implementing adequate
internal controls (e.g., Annas, 1989; Ennis & Emery, 1978; Szasz,
1975). These advocates note that the actions of health professionals
are naturally shielded from view by the fiduciary and confidential elements of the treatment alliance. Therefore, they believe it is essential
to enhance society's view into the interstices of the therapeutic interaction (e.g., Bach, 1989; Bersoff, 1992; Heimberg, 1983; Klugman,
1983; Saks, 1986; Weithorn, 1988).

Both sides of the debate point to legal precedent to support their
conclusions about the current level of oversight. In order to reconcile

this precedent, it is necessary to recognize a distinction between the *substantive* and *procedural* elements of law. The degree of deference shown to clinical decision making depends on which component is implicated. Substantive legal criteria are defined by constitution, statute, regulation, or case law, and cannot be ignored or altered. However, practically speaking, there is considerable latitude in establishing the procedures for resolving legal issues. By granting health professionals the power to apply legal standards, the courts and legislatures have, in effect, adopted a hands-off approach, deferring to professional judgment except in the most egregious cases. Consider the following vignette, which parallels facts from a U.S. Supreme Court case:

> Hospital is a 500-bed, state-subsidized health-care facility in State A. Larry Lawyer filed a civil action against Hospital's superintendent and several members of the attending staff, alleging that the defendants violated the civil rights of Mr. Stuck, a former patient who was involuntarily confined to the psychiatric service for two months. The hospital superintendent had continuously rejected Mr. Stuck's pleas for release, stating that "continued milieu therapy is in his best interests." The relevant state statute contained no provisions for review of the propriety of such confinements.

> Following a trial on the merits, the court held that the defendants' actions violated the plaintiff's liberty interest, and held them liable for damages in tort. The following morning, the local newspaper quoted Hospital's attorney as stating that "the court's holding was an unacceptable incursion into the province of health-care professionals. Now, every mental health professional must worry about how her decisions will be perceived in hindsight. Of course, we're going to appeal."

On similar facts, the U.S. Supreme Court held that such actions by hospital personnel are unconstitutional, and that, at a minimum, a finding of dangerousness or inability to survive safely in the community is required for involuntary civil commitment (*O'Connor v. Donaldson*, 1975). However, contrary to the allegations of Hospital's attorney, this decision was a very limited incursion into the health-care domain, and represented an explicit compromise between the needs for autonomy of health-care professionals and for judicial review of potential abuses.

As noted, legal decisions have substantive and procedural components, and the appropriate degree of judicial deference depends on which component is implicated. The *O'Connor* decision stands for two independent propositions: (1) individuals cannot be deprived of liberty in the absence of a threshold showing of "dangerousness," and (2) mental health professionals cannot act in an arbitrary and unreviewable manner. The first proposition reflects a substantive legal standard. It is clearly the province of the courts to discern and define such criteria. The second proposition relates to the procedures that must be followed in establishing whether the substantive criteria have been satisfied. Notably, the *O'Connor* court never answered the questions of whether the determination of "dangerousness" can be made by mental health professionals and of what procedures must be followed. The Court merely held that some form of minimum determination, based on definable criteria, is constitutionally mandated.

The *O'Connor* decision was predicated on the U.S. Constitution. In our federal system of government, the Constitution defines the minimum protections available. It is possible for state laws to create or define broader substantive rights. State courts and legislatures, however, typically have refused to do so, preferring to defer to the judgments of health practitioners. For example, New York's Mental Hygiene Law (1988 & Supp. 1991, secs. 9.01, 9.27) provides that a mentally ill individual may be involuntarily committed if, in the opinions of two certifying physicians and the hospital's medical director, care and treatment are "essential to such person's welfare." This is clearly a vague and minimalist interpretation of the *O'Connor* "dangerousness" requirement.

*O'Connor* also appears to define both the minimum and maximum procedural protections available. Consider the following composite vignette:

Delighted over his recent victory against Hospital, Larry Lawyer decided to bring two new actions against the facility. The first complaint charges that the hospital violated the liberty interests of Ralph Runaway, a 13-year-old boy whose mother had him involuntarily committed to the adolescent service. Ralph's parents are divorced, and he never knew his father. His mother is a chronic alcoholic, who has been treated on a voluntary basis at Hospital for dysthymia and personality disorder NOS. She states that Ralph is incorrigible because he keeps leaving home and school to search for his father and to play video games. It appears that her petition was motivated by her need for peace and quiet in the home, as her nerves have been particularly shot recently. Doctor Do-Good interviewed Ralph for less than 10 minutes, and he concluded that he was "suitable" for treatment.

In *Parham v. J.R.* (1979), the U.S. Supreme Court addressed the issue of the procedural due process rights of minor children whose guardians sought institutionalized mental health treatment for them. The Court acknowledged that the Constitution gives citizens (including minors) the right to antecedent, independent review by a "neutral magistrate" prior to infringement of the fundamental right of liberty. Notably, however, the Court held that this inquiry was best left to medical and mental health professionals.

> Due process has never been thought to require that the neutral and detached trier of fact be law trained or a judicial or administrative officer. Surely, this is the case as to medical decisions, for neither judges nor administrative hearing officers are better qualified than psychiatrists to render psychiatric judgments. Thus, a staff physician will suffice, so long as he or she is free to evaluate independently the child's mental and emotional condition and need for treatment.
>
> It is not necessary that the deciding physician conduct a formal or quasi-formal hearing. A state is free to require such a hearing, but due process is not violated by use of informal, traditional medical investigative techniques. (p. 607 [citations omitted])

Similarly, in *Washington v. Harper* (1990), the Supreme Court held that due process is not violated where correctional inmates are subjected to involuntary treatment with psychotropic medication or other intrusive procedures without the benefit of independent review by a judicial magistrate. The Court held that the Constitution permits medical personnel to make the decision under "fair procedural mechanisms" (p. 1042).

Notably, in the above vignette, it is apparently of little consequence that the petition for commitment was motivated by Ralph's mother's personal problems. Although there is considerable debate about whether parents always act in the best interests of their children and whether inpatient treatment is appropriate for minors (Weithorn, 1988), the Court was unwilling to take these concerns at face value. In effect, the Court deferred to health-care professionals to assess the degree of family dysfunction and the suitability of hospitalizing the identified patient.

These cases place direct responsibility for evaluating and safeguarding fundamental liberty interests into the hands of health-care professionals, thus creating, in effect, a new class of de facto magistrates. And it would be erroneous to conclude that they are limited on their facts to less protected classes of citizens, such as minors and prison inmates. Consider the following:

Larry Lawyer's second complaint concerns Mr. Cronic, a 45-year-old man who has been at Hospital for 10 months. Mr. Cronic has carried a diagnosis of schizophrenia since his first break at age 20. Based on psychological testing, his I.Q. is estimated to be in the borderline to deficient range, and he appears to have a learning disability. While at Hospital, Mr. Cronic has been treated with a variety of neuroleptic medications by various medical residents and fellows doing six-week rotations on his unit. He has also been involved in several behavior modification programs designed to increase his socialization and to contain his "inappropriate intrusiveness." These programs were implemented by creative art therapy students from a neighboring college. Mr. Cronic's parents have repeatedly requested that he be treated by a certified psychoanalyst, but their pleas have been ignored.

In *Youngberg v. Romeo* (1982), the Supreme Court addressed the constitutional rights of mental health inpatients. Although dubbed a "right to treatment" case, it provides almost no discernible rights at all. The *Youngberg* Court held that institutionalized patients have a substantive due process right to minimally adequate or reasonable habilitation to ensure their safety and freedom from undue restraint. Recognizing that this necessitates individualized, fact-sensitive determinations, the Court had to decide how and by whom those determinations were to be made. Reasoning that judges and juries are no better qualified than health professionals to make such judgments, the Court left the procedural mechanism in the hands of those professionals, subject to minimal oversight:

> [T]he decision, if made by a professional, is presumptively valid; liability may be imposed only when the decision by the professional is such a substantial departure from accepted professional judgment, practice, or standards as to demonstrate that the person responsible actually did not base the decision on such a judgment. (p. 323)

There is simply no lesser standard of judicial review than that articulated in *Youngberg*. The professional's decision must be so illogical, arbitrary, or vague as to, in effect, constitute no decision at all (see also *Society for Good Will to Retarded Children v. Cuomo*, 1990).

*Youngberg* was based on a federal constitutional theory. It should be noted that other avenues of redress are available to patients, and some of these do not require government action or complicity to establish liability. For example, many state legislatures have passed "patient bill of rights" statutes (e.g., New York Mental Hygiene Law, 1988 & Supp. 1991, secs. 33.01 *et seq.*), which create enforceable standards of care. Similarly, efforts have been made to find enhanced protection in such federal statutes as Section 504 of the Rehabilitation Act (1973) and the Developmentally Disabled Assistance and Bill of Rights Act (1975) (see, e.g., *Pennhurst State School and Hospital v. Halderman*, 1984). Notably, however, such statutory safeguards are typically directed to the hospital environment or milieu, as opposed to the content of patient care. The provisions address such issues as the patients' right to privacy, the free practice of religion, safe and sanitary conditions, nutritious meals, and freedom from abuse.

Patients can also bring malpractice or tort actions against clinicians if the provision of services falls below the "generally accepted" professional standard of care, which is a higher standard than that enunciated in *Youngberg*. Clearly, malpractice actions are a significant source of concern (and rage) for health-care professionals (e.g., Bennett et al., 1990). This concern has taken on greater intensity in light of the recent specter of "right to *effective* treatment" cases.

In the controversial *Osheroff v. Chestnut Lodge* litigation (see Klerman, 1990; Stone, 1990), the plaintiff alleged that it was malpractice for the defendants to treat him solely with psychoanalytically oriented psychotherapy and to fail to institute pharmacotherapy for his major depressive symptoms. The case ended in an undisclosed, out-of-court settlement, but it raised many important questions, not the least of which was the relative roles of law and science. Are courts and juries qualified to evaluate conflicting scientific philosophies about diagnosis and treatment and to weigh contrary empirical data? For example, is Mr. Cronic in the above vignette entitled to psychoanalysis or to treatment by seasoned professionals as opposed to treatment by students and trainees?

Attempts at prediction are always precarious, but it is unlikely that courts will allow nonscientists to make these decisions. Divergent legal theories do not alter the practical implications of allowing laypersons to review the activities of professionals. The Supreme Court's conclusion that judges and juries are not qualified to make health-care decisions should not change merely because an action is based on malpractice rather than constitutional law. It is likely that the courts will continue to enforce the kinds of obligations contained in patients' bill-of-rights statutes, which are directed at the therapeutic milieu, and to defer to health-care professionals on matters of treatment.

In those cases where courts endorse specific forms of treatment, the contours of accepted practice are discerned from explicit institutional and industry standards, such as professional ethical codes, Joint Commission on Accreditation of Healthcare Organizations (JCAHO) guidelines, quality assurance standards, and institutional bylaws (see *Darling v. Charleston Community Memorial Hospital*, 1966; *Purcell v.*

*Zimbelman,* 1972). In these cases, the courts are merely taking judicial notice of generally accepted practice, rather than substituting their judgment for that of health-care practitioners (Curran & Shapiro, 1982).

## Limitations of Deference to Professionals' Procedures

Generally speaking, courts and legislatures have given significant responsibility and authority for vindicating fundamental legal interests to health-care professionals, investing them with de facto judicial powers. This new class of "magistrates" apparently has the authority to establish the procedures by which substantive rights are to be enforced. Notably, however, this broad authority is curtailed in two ways: (1) the procedures are subject to the *O'Connor* requirements of reviewability and nonarbitrariness, and (2) health-care professionals cannot ignore or redefine substantive rights. Consider the following:

> Larry Lawyer recently filed another action against Hospital's admissions and emergency room staffs on behalf of Mr. Cloud, a chronic substance abuser who has suffered several small strokes as the result of cocaine use. Extensive neuropsychological testing administered during a prior stay at Hospital revealed that Mr. Cloud has a mild multi-infarct dementia, characterized by deficits in short-term memory and moderate spatial disorientation. Approximately one month earlier, Mr. Cloud walked into Hospital's emergency room in an obviously intoxicated condition. He was oriented to person and partially to place, but not to time, and he seemed to be having tactile hallucinations of bugs on his skin. He was deficient on serial sevens and digits forward and backward. Eager to relieve Mr. Cloud's obvious torment, Dr. Rapid had him sign a voluntary admission form (as he had done many times before), and personally escorted him to the addictions section of the adult psychiatric unit.

In *Zinermon v. Burch* (1990), the Supreme Court held that hospital personnel violated the procedural due process rights of a patient who entered their facility on a voluntary status because the patient signed the admission consent form while in a disoriented state and may have been incompetent to give informed consent. The Court held that, although it may be permissible for mental health professionals to make the determination of competence to consent to treatment, there must be some form of fair procedural mechanism in place.

[The State] chose to delegate to petitioners a broad power to admit patients to [the hospital] . . . . Because petitioners had state authority to deprive persons of liberty, the Constitution imposed on them the State's concomitant duty to see that no deprivations occur without adequate procedural protections. (p. 988)

Significantly, *Zinermon* does not stand for the proposition that the courts may override the conclusions of mental health professionals. Presumably, if the defendants had made an explicit determination, following reasonable medical procedures, that the plaintiff was competent to consent, there would have been no liability. The fault of the defendants was that they made no determination at all, and that they had no procedure available for making such a determination. The Court was concerned that these officials should be held accountable for the "abuse of their *broadly delegated, uncircumscribed power* to effect the deprivation at issue" (p. 989 [emphasis added]). The actions of mental health professionals must be reviewable and nonarbitrary.

Upon admission to the addictions unit, Mr. Cloud changed his mind about treatment and became increasingly anxious and agitated. He refused all medications, and was unresponsive to efforts by the nursing staff to engage him in conversation or unit activities. He continuously rocked back and forth in front of the TV in the community room, and refused to go to sleep. Eager to relieve his obvious torment, Dr. Rapid ordered an involuntary sedative injection, reasoning that Mr. Cloud was obviously incompetent to make a treatment decision. Prior to giving the order, Dr. Rapid conferred with the medical director of Hospital, who agreed that Mr. Cloud was incompetent to refuse treatment.

Patients have a substantive due process right to refuse medical treatment, which can be overridden in only two instances (*Mills v.*

*Rogers,* 1982; see Note, 1990; *Rivers v. Katz,* 1986). First, pursuant to the State's *police power,* it is permissible to medicate a patient involuntarily when he or she presents an immediate danger to self or others. The authority to administer such treatment is justified only for as long as the emergency continues. Considering the risk involved, health-care personnel are given substantial discretion to define what constitutes an "emergency," and the procedural mechanisms for making the determination may be quite informal.

Second, pursuant to the *parens patriae* (state paternalism) power, it is permissible to treat a patient involuntarily to prevent a deterioration in his or her condition. Notably, unlike the emergency situation, this justification requires that the patient be incompetent to choose for himself or herself. Significantly, "competence" is a substantive legal standard, which, as noted previously, cannot be ignored or redefined by mental health professionals. In the absence of an emergency, Dr. Rapid's and the medical director's presumption of incompetence without formal inquiry is insufficient. It is incumbent on them to apply the relevant statutory definition of "competency" (e.g., New York Mental Hygiene Law, 1988 & Supp. 1991, secs. 78.01 *et seq.*) prior to reaching a conclusion. Depending on the state, following an internal, administrative determination of incompetency, the patient may also have the right of de novo review by a court (see *Rivers v. Katz,* 1986).

## TRANSLATING SUBSTANTIVE LEGAL CRITERIA INTO PSYCHOLEGAL CONSTRUCTS

As the previous vignette points out, although mental health professionals have substantial authority to evaluate fundamental interests, they are required to apply substantive legal criteria. This frequently poses a dilemma for these professionals, as they are not legally trained (Horowitz & Willging, 1984, Chap. 2), and as legal concepts often do not have immediately discernible scientific counterparts (Marlowe, 1988; Melton, Petrila, Poythress, & Slobogin, 1987). It is, therefore, necessary for clinicians operationally to define or translate legal concepts into observable, definable, and measurable scientific terms (Grisso, 1986). These "psycholegal" constructs cannot supplant or alter legal criteria, but they can serve to reformulate them in a usable manner.

It is beyond the scope of this chapter—and, indeed, this book—to address the extensive number of psycholegal constructs that are required in general clinical practice. However, preliminary translations of two prominent legal concepts are provided in order to illustrate the process of psycholegal reformulation.

## A Psycholegal Formulation of Competence

Ms. Senil is a 96-year-old widow who underwent surgery at Hospital for a severe hernia. When she regained consciousness, her doctors noticed a change in her mental status. Her mood seemed uncharacteristically belligerent. She was forgetful, and occasionally appeared to be responding to people and events from a remote time in her life. Hospital's social-work team concluded that she should be transferred to a nearby nursing facility because she was no longer able to care for herself adequately. After much cajoling, Ms. Senil agreed to the transfer. However, the team is unsure whether she is competent to give informed consent to the transfer and, despite extensive efforts, has been unable to locate any of her relatives. The team requested a consultation with Dr. Law of the consultation–liaison service, who concluded that (1) Ms. Senil is suffering from an "irreversible dementia of unknown origin," (2) she is unable to perform daily chores, (3) she understands the nature and consequences of the decision before her, and (4) she is "clearly making the right decision."

"Incompetence" is a legal conclusion—as opposed to a psychiatric diagnosis—and can only be determined by a duly appointed legal authority. Clinicians therefore may assume that this issue does not concern them, since all they can do is file a petition to commence a judicial proceeding (e.g., New York Mental Hygiene Law, sec. 78.03). However, consider what would happen if Dr. Law were to conclude summarily that Ms. Senil was competent. A formal determination would not be triggered, and, as Ms. Senil had agreed to the transfer and has no relatives to contest it, it is unlikely that the decision would be challenged. In effect, a failure to raise the issue would be tantamount to a determination of competence. Further, courts are notorious for "rubber-stamping" the conclusions of experts on matters that appear to be predominantly "medical" in nature. In order for a court to evaluate the evidence fairly, it is necessary for experts to operationalize the statutory criteria.

From a psycholegal perspective, statutory definitions of incompetence vary along three dimensions. Depending on the jurisdiction, incompetence may be defined as reflecting (1) specific disorders or disabilities, (2) an impairment in decision-making or communication abilities, (3) an impairment in functional abilities, or (4) some combination of these (Anderer, 1990). For example, New York (Mental Hygiene Law, sec. 78.01) defines an individual as incompetent if "by reason of advanced age, illness, infirmity, mental weakness, alcohol abuse, addiction to drugs, or other cause, [he] has suffered substantial impairment of his ability to care for his property or has become unable to provide for himself or others dependent upon him for support . . . ." This statute combines a nonexclusive list of disabilities with generalized functional impairment.

Assuming that the statute in State A addresses all three dimensions of competence, Dr. Law's conclusions would implicate each of those components. Her diagnosis of dementia, for example, implicates the first prong, relating to the presence of a disorder. Her conclusion that Ms. Senil cannot perform daily chores is an example of functional impairment, while her conclusion that Ms. Senil understands the nature and consequences of the decision suggests an absence of impairment in her decision-making and communication abilities. What, then, should Dr. Law conclude?

Generally, there is a judicial and legislative preference for a determination of partial incompetency, as opposed to an assumption of general incapacitation (Anderer, 1990). Thus Dr. Law's conclusion that Ms. Senil is unable to perform daily chores does not imply that she cannot make decisions and plan rationally for her care. She can be incompetent to cook and clean, while fully competent to manage her finances, write a will, and choose a home.

The ability to reach a workable decision, and to communicate that decision to others, appears to be at the heart of the psycholegal formulation of competence (Tepper & Elwork, 1984). However, there are many ways to evaluate a decision. For example, the clinician could focus solely on the presence or absence of an expression of will, avoiding a value judgment as to the utility of the result. In contrast, the clinician could attempt to evaluate the rationality of the outcome by, for example, considering what percentage of individuals make such a decision.

The problem with defining competence in these ways is that the clinician risks tolerating an irrational decision or introducing personal bias into the process. It is therefore preferable to concentrate on the decision-making *process* and the subject's awareness of the contours of the dilemma; that is (Tepper & Elwork, 1984): Did the subject consider a sufficient range of objectives and alternative courses of action? Did she weigh the costs and benefits of each alternative? Did she search for essential or important missing information? Did she reexamine the alternatives in light of this new information? Did she plan and make adequate provisions for implementing the chosen course of action? By operationalizing "competency" in this manner, clinicians' "interrater reliability" will be vastly improved, thus diminishing the embarrassingly inconsistent conclusions that have been reached by mental health professionals in the past.

## A Psycholegal Formulation of Autonomy

Unfortunately, the sedative that was administered to Mr. Cloud [earlier vignette] did not have its intended effect. He became increasingly paranoid after being injected with what he perceived to be "poison to the mind." He began pacing in an agitated state and glaring menacingly at the staff and fellow patients. When the occupational therapist asked him if he wanted to make a collage with her, he threw a chair against the wall. Ima Incharge, RN, confronted Mr. Cloud, informing him that if he didn't immediately cease his unacceptable and intolerable behavior, he would be forcibly escorted to the quiet room. Mr. Cloud responded that he didn't have to listen to anybody, that she wasn't his mother, and that he was all-powerful. Nurse Incharge, unimpressed by Mr. Cloud's reported powers, carried him to the seclusion room and placed him in four-point restraint.

Upon hearing of this, Larry Lawyer appended a new count to his complaint on behalf of Mr. Cloud, alleging that the restraint violated his rights to liberty and autonomy. In her answer to the complaint, Nurse Incharge explained that restraints are therapeutic for disorganized patients, providing them with assurance that they will not be allowed to lose control and serving to shore up diffuse ego boundaries. And, in any event, it was necessary for the safety of the ward.

Traditionally, the courts have viewed restraint and seclusion as little different from other forms of treatment or unit management, and have left their regulation to internal professional norms (Saks, 1986; see *Youngberg v. Romeo,* 1982). More recently, patients' bill-of-rights statutes have addressed the issue directly, but the level of oversight varies considerably. For example, some states require only that the episode and rationale for restraint be recorded, while others require that it be ordered by designated authorities. Other states specify the conditions under which restraint may be implemented, that is, dangerousness or medical necessity (see Saks, 1986, p. 1841, n. 25). Typically, the statutes also address the mechanics of restraint, required monitoring practices, care of the patient, and renewal of orders (see New York Mental Hygiene Law, sec. 33.04).

Even where the relevant statute requires an antecedent finding of "dangerousness" or "medical necessity," those terms are sufficiently vague and flexible to give considerable authority and discretion to health-care practitioners. It is, therefore, incumbent on clinicians to operationalize the concept of autonomy, as well as its counterweights, in order to give it practical meaning and effect (see generally Anderer, 1992).

A competency determination presumes that a rational patient could choose either of several alternative courses of action, and it is the *process* of reaching the decision that is the focus of attention. However, in certain instances, a particular course of action is unacceptable, regardless of the process by which the decision is reached. For instance, it is unacceptable for Mr. Cloud to endanger other individuals, regardless of how or why he chooses to do so. This limited class of cases— termed "emergency situations"—justifies interventions that restrict patients' physical liberty and autonomy. As noted earlier, the intervention is justified only for as long as the emergency continues. Further, because of the immediate risk of danger, significant deference is accorded health professionals to define the nature and extent of the risk.

Restrictions on autonomy are also justified in a second class of cases. Assume, for example, that Mr. Cloud deeply desired to go to his room, but, because of the nature of his illness, he was unable to comply. Nurse Incharge alluded to this issue in her explanation of external ego boundaries. In such circumstances, the staff's intervention is aimed at helping Mr. Cloud attain his own goal, and is not legally or ethically objectionable. In effect, there is no infringement on autonomy.

The difficulty, of course, is in ascertaining what Mr. Cloud's goals are, or will be after his illness subsides. There is always the danger that health professionals will substitute their own goals for those of the patient, and rationalize their interventions after the fact. Therefore, in this second class of cases, it is necessary for the patient's wishes to be reliably and clearly expressed, so that the staff's actions can be judged against some external criterion.

Notably, it is this analysis that underlay the Supreme Court's decision recognizing the right of terminally ill patients to terminate life-sustaining treatments (*Cruzan v. Missouri Department of Health,* 1990). The Court held that the family of a comatose person may carry out the patient's desire to cease treatment, but only if the patient's wishes have been reliably and clearly expressed.

In these types of cases, the burden is on the health-care professional to establish the patient's true intent, and the professional is required to point to explicit statements or behaviors by the patient that manifested this intent. In the case of Mr. Cloud, no such behaviors were manifested. However, assume that he stated that voices were confusing him, and that he felt too high and anxious to sit still. Under such circumstances, it could reasonably be inferred that he desired containment. Given the courts' willingness to defer to health professionals, this conclusion would likely be upheld.

The psycholegal formulation of autonomy involves an assessment of a patient's ability to understand directions and to contain his or her behavior within the specified boundaries. This implicates familiar elements of mental status, such as impulse control, delay of gratification, affect and mood stability, reality testing, sensorium, and psychomotor control. Further, mental health professionals are expert at observing behavior, and these observational skills are essential for establishing whether the patient communicated a desire to be contained or directed in a given manner.

These formulations of "competence" and "autonomy" are highly cursory, and they do not go far in highlighting the extensive list of psycholegal constructs that are required in clinical practice. The goals of this book are to begin this process of psycholegal reformulation and to help create a vocabulary for the process. The following chapters are organized by treatment contexts and issues, to identify the prominent psycholegal issues presented in various settings.

## REFERENCES

Anderer, S. J. (1990). *Determining competency in guardianship proceedings* (Public Service Monograph Series No. 1). Washington, DC: American Bar Association.

Anderer, S. J. (Ed.). (1992). Integrating legal and psychological perspectives on the right to personal autonomy. [symposium issue]. *Villanova Law Review, 37* (6).

Annas, G. J. (1989). *The rights of hospital patients* (2d ed.). Carbondale, IL: Southern Illinois University Press.

Bach, J. P. (1989). Requiring due care in the process of patient deinstitutionalization: Toward a common law approach to mental health care reform. *Yale Law Journal, 98,* 1153–1172.

Bennett, B. E., Bryant, B. K., VandenBos, G. R., & Greenwood, A. (1990). *Professional liability and risk management.* Washington, DC: American Psychological Association.

Bersoff, D. N. (1992). Autonomy for vulnerable populations: The Supreme Court's reckless disregard for self-determination and social science. *Villanova Law Review, 37,* 1569–1605.

*Cruzan v. Missouri Department of Health,* 110 S.Ct. 2841 (1990).

Curran, W. J., & Shapiro, E. D. (1982). *Law, medicine and forensic science.* Boston, MA: Little, Brown.

*Darling v. Charleston Community Memorial Hospital,* 33 Ill.2d 326, 211 N.E.2d 253 (1965), *cert. denied,* 383 U.S. 946 (1966).

Developmentally Disabled Assistance and Bill of Rights Act of 1975, Pub. L, No. 94-103, 489 Stat. 496, *codified at* 42 U.S.C. secs. 6001 *et seq.*

Ennis, B. J., & Emery, R. (1978). *The rights of mental patients* (rev. ed.). New York: Avon.

Everstine, L., & Everstine, D. S. (Eds.). (1986). *Psychotherapy and the law.* Orlando, FL: Grune & Stratton.

Grisso, T. (1986). *Evaluating competencies: Forensic assessments and instruments.* New York: Plenum.

Heimberg, S. A. (1983). Status of the emergency room psychotherapist: Privacy rites. *UCLA Law Review, 30,* 1317–1348.

Horowitz, I. A., & Willging, T. E. (1984). *The psychology of law: Integrations and applications.* Boston, MA: Little, Brown.

Klerman, G. L. (1990). The psychiatric patient's right to effective treatment: Implications of *Osheroff v. Chestnut Lodge. American Journal of Psychiatry, 147,* 409–418.

Klugman, E. (1983). Toward a uniform right to medical records: A proposal for a model patient access and information practices statute. *UCLA Law Review, 30,* 1349–1377.

Marlowe, D. B. (1988). Negligent infliction of mental distress: A jurisdictional survey of existing limitation devices and proposal based on an analysis of objective versus subjective indices of distress. *Villanova Law Review, 33,* 781–833.

Melton, G. B., Petrila, J., Poythress, N. G., & Slobogin, C. (1987). *Psychological evaluations for the courts.* New York: Guilford.

Miller, R. D. (1986). *Problems in hospital law* (5th ed.). Rockville, MD: Aspen.

*Mills v. Rogers,* 457 U.S. 291 (1982), *vacating sub. nom., Rogers v. Okin.* 634 F.2d 650 (1st Cir. 1980); *on remand,* 738 F.2d 1 (1st Cir. 1984).

New York Mental Hygiene Law, secs. 9.01 *et seq.;* 33.01 *et seq.;* 77.01 *et seq.;* 78.01 *et seq.* (McKinney, 1988 & Supp. 1991).

Note (1990). Developments in the law: Medical technology and the law. *Harvard Law Review, 103,* 1519–1676.

*O'Connor v. Donaldson,* 422 U.S. 563 (1975).

*Parham v. J.R.,* 442 U.S. 584 (1979).

*Pennhurst State School and Hospital v. Halderman,* 465 U.S. 89 (1984), *reversing,* 673 F.2d 647 (3d Cir. 1982).

*Purcell v. Zimbelman,* 18 Ariz. App. 75, 500 P.2d 335 (1972).

Rehabilitation Act of 1973, sec. 504, 87 Stat. 394, *codified at* 29 U.S.C. sec. 794.

*Rivers v. Katz,* 67 N.Y.2d 485, 495 N.E.2d 337 (1986).

Saks, E. R. (1986). The use of mechanical restraints in psychiatric hospitals. *Yale Law Journal, 95,* 1836–1856.

*Society for Good Will to Retarded Children v. Cuomo,* 902 F.2d 1085 (2d Cir. 1990).

Stone, A. A. (1990). Law, science, and psychiatric malpractice: A response to Klerman's indictment of psychoanalytic psychiatry. *American Journal of Psychiatry, 147,* 419–427.

Szasz, T. S. (1975). The danger of coercive psychiatry. *American Bar Association Journal, 61,* 1246–1248.

Tepper, A. M., & Elwork, A. (1984). Competence to consent to treatment as a psycholegal construct. *Law and Human Behavior, 8,* 205–223.

*Washington v. Harper,* 110 S.Ct. 1028 (1990).

Weithorn, L. A. (1988). Mental hospitalization of troublesome youth: An analysis of skyrocketing admission rates. *Stanford Law Review, 40,* 773–838.

*Youngberg v. Romeo,* 457 U.S. 307 (1982).

*Zinermon v. Burch,* 110 S.Ct. 975 (1990).

# 2

## Ethics and Decision Making in Psychiatric Practice in General Hospitals

RUTH MACKLIN

### ETHICS AND LAW IN CLINICAL PRACTICE

Law and ethics overlap in psychiatric practice, as they do in the broader social arena. Many laws have an underlying ethical rationale, and existing laws can be repealed or modified when they are evaluated from an ethical point of view. For example, laws that authorized racially segregated facilities were overturned during the civil rights movement, when equal rights for blacks were officially recognized and when it was demonstrated that schools could not be both separate and equal. Law and ethics are intertwined in such prominent concepts as privacy and confidentiality, individual liberty, personal autonomy, protecting the public from risk of harm, and preventing individuals from harming themselves. Decision making by mental health professionals in general hospitals thus encompasses both legal and ethical elements.

It is sometimes thought that laws give clear guidance, while ethics is a fuzzy discipline, fraught with uncertainty and differing subjective opinions about right and wrong. That view errs in both directions. It presumes too much in the way of certainty arising out of court decisions and statutory law, and it accords too little weight to the application of settled ethical principles. This chapter explores issues at the intersection of ethics, psychiatry, and law as they arise in clinical practice in the general hospital. Ethical dilemmas can result

21

from uncertainty about facts or probabilities, differing ethical priorities, or ambiguities in the law. Problems can also occur when ethical principles come into conflict, when potentially applicable legal principles clash, or when mental health professionals perceive a need to balance their own personal interests against those of their patients.

## Informed Consent and Treatment Refusals

One of the most common situations facing psychiatrists in the general hospital is that of patients who refuse medical treatments. Although patients' refusals of treatment are usually troubling to physicians, such refusals are not always irrational. Nevertheless, patients who resist recommended therapy are frequently viewed as irrational, and so a physician or surgeon typically calls for a psychiatric consultation to assess the patient's capacity to make medical decisions.

Not surprisingly, the capacity of patients who go along willingly with their doctors' recommendations is rarely questioned, despite the fact that permission for invasive procedures is routinely granted by patients whose mental capacity is impaired as a result of psychiatric illness, dementia, delirium, or other causes. Failure to question a patient's consent to treatment is understandable from a medical perspective, and might even be justifiable from an ethical point of view. If the proposed medical treatment will truly benefit the patient, proceeding with therapy is likely to result in more good than harm, whereas foregoing the treatment is likely to have a bad outcome.

This asymmetry—questioning the capacity of patients who refuse treatment and presuming the competence of those who consent—is also troubling from another standpoint. The ethical premise underlying the doctrine of informed consent is that the patient has a right to self-determination in the medical setting. Just as people enjoy the right to liberty and autonomy (so long as they abide by the law) in everyday life, so, too, in the medical setting patients have a moral and legal right to determine what may be done to them. The singular exception is that of patients who lack the capacity to decide for themselves, a circumstance that usually gives rise to a psychiatric consultation.

Decisional capacity is generally referred to as "competency" in the medical setting, but the concept of competency is a legal as well as a psychological one (Roth, Meisel, & Lidz, 1977). Strictly speaking, the determination of incompetency is a judicial matter, one that can be made only by a judge. However, judicial determinations usually rely on recommendations by psychiatrists following an evaluation of the patient.

An early statement of the legal doctrine of informed consent was articulated by Justice Benjamin Cardozo in a landmark case in 1914. Cardozo's statement embodied both the right to self-determination and the singular exception: "Every human being of adult years and sound mind has a right to determine what shall be done with his own body . . ." (*Schloendorff v. New York Hospital,* 1914, 211 N.Y. at 129). Although this legal and ethical principle is clear, it can be difficult to apply. For consent to be properly informed, patients must have the ability to understand the information presented, and pertinent information must be conveyed in nontechnical language at a level commensurate with the patient's actual capacity to understand. Therefore, if the doctrine of informed consent is to be meaningful, it is crucial that patients' decisional capacity be accurately assessed.

## PRINCIPLES OF BIOMEDICAL ETHICS

Both the right of patients to grant voluntary, informed consent to treatment and the corresponding desire of physicians to override patients' refusal of recommended treatments are supported by respected ethical principles. The bioethical principle that underlies the need to obtain informed consent is respect for autonomy: "Autonomous actions are not to be subjected to controlling constraints by others" (Beauchamp & Childress, 1989, p. 72). This principle permits a patient who acts autonomously to refuse a medical treatment even if that treatment promises to provide some benefit. Accordingly, the principle directs the physician to respect the autonomy of the patient.

From the physician's perspective, a different ethical principle stands in the forefront. That principle is sometimes stated in the form of the ancient precept of medical ethics, "Do no harm." In the parlance of contemporary bioethics it is known as the principle of nonmaleficence: One ought not to inflict evil or harm (Beauchamp & Childress, 1989, p. 122). However, the injunction to "do no harm" operates more as a slogan than as a moral principle capable of giving guidance for decision making. Any medical intervention is bound to cause some harm to a patient—pain, side effects from drugs, loss of blood. The goal of medical treatment is to bring about more good than harm, a balance of more good consequences than potentially bad ones. Thus a formulation of the ethical imperative to physicians that is preferable to nonmaleficence ("Do no harm") is stated in the principle of beneficence. This ethical principle has three variations (Beauchamp & Childress, 1989, p. 123): (1) one ought to prevent evil or harm, (2) one ought to remove evil or harm, (3) one ought to do or promote good. These variations can be collapsed into the single proposition: One ought to strive to bring about a balance of beneficial consequences over harmful ones.

Situations in which patients refuse recommended therapy typically give rise to a conflict between these two leading ethical principles. The principle of respect for autonomy grants patients the right to self-determination, including the refusal of medical treatment, and requires that physicians respect their patients' autonomy. But the principle of beneficence enjoins physicians to bring about the best outcomes for their patients, which presumably entails administering the therapy. It is not possible to adhere to both ethical principles simultaneously, and so an ethical dilemma results. In the face of an ethical dilemma arising out of a conflict of principles, two strategies are open to the decision maker. One strategy is to choose one of the two conflicting principles to act on, and then seek to justify that choice. The other strategy is to try to escape between the horns of the dilemma.

The problem with the first strategy is that decision makers tend to choose their preferred principle on the basis of preexisting values, and then to construct a rationale for choosing that principle. For health professionals, the preferred principle will almost always be beneficence. Everything in the training of psychiatrists and other health professionals directs them to seek the best therapeutic outcomes for their patients. Conversely, patients (or their advocates) will typically assert their decision-making autonomy, justified by the claim that it is their right to determine what shall happen to their bodies ("Whose life is it, anyway?").

The prevailing view in bioethics is that the principle of respect for autonomy takes precedence over the principle of beneficence, thereby granting patients the ultimate authority to decide for themselves. That view is buttressed by several lines of judicial decisions, which include granting medically ill patients the right to forgo life-sustaining therapy, giving psychiatric patients the right to refuse psychoactive medications, and recognizing the validity of advance directives in the form of a living will or the appointment of a health-care proxy.

The second strategy, attempting to escape between the horns of the dilemma, is adopted when physicians question the capacity of patients to exercise their autonomy properly. A complicating factor in applying the respect-for-autonomy principle is that sick people sometimes lack decisional capacity. Competence is a precondition of being able to decide or act autonomously (Beauchamp & Childress, 1989, p. 79). The principle of respect for autonomy thus has a corollary, which rests on the widely recognized ethical conviction that "persons with diminished autonomy are entitled to protection" (National Commission for the Protection of Human Subjects, 1979, p. 4). Acknowledging the validity of the principle of respect for autonomy does not rule out recognizing specific exceptions, cases in which freedom of choice and action may be curtailed. These exceptions comprise a range of justified acts of paternalism—acting for the good or benefit of individuals with diminished autonomy, even in the absence of their explicit consent.

The paradigm of justified paternalism is restricting the freedom of small children for their own good. Not only are such restrictions permitted ethically, but they are ethically obligatory. However, when does a child attain sufficient autonomy to warrant freedom from parental or other controls? Since the acquisition of full autonomy is a gradual process, decisions need to be made about the circumstances in which paternalism ceases to be justifiable. Similar problems arise with respect to another population with diminished autonomy: mentally retarded persons. Profoundly mentally retarded persons lack the cognitive ability to make judgments about their own safety, and so paternalistic interference and restriction are justified for this group. But what about the mildly mentally retarded?

These line-drawing issues are equally problematic in the case of psychiatric patients. The types of psychiatric disorders are too numerous and varied to allow a simple answer to the question of when paternalism can be ethically justified. The mere fact of a psychiatric diagnosis is not an automatic presumption of a patient's lack of competence, so psychiatric patients retain the right to autonomous decision making until a determination is made that they are incompetent. Although it is widely held that persons with diminished capacity stand in need of protection, disagreements begin at the point where assessments have to be made. What is the criterion for "full" autonomy? How far short of full autonomy warrants overriding an individual's decisions? These uncertainties create problems for psychiatric consultants when they are called by their medical colleagues to evaluate a patient's capacity to give an informed refusal of treatment.

Both the principle of respect for autonomy and that of beneficence are accepted as valid ethical principles. No problem arises in their application when each is taken by itself. Ethical dilemmas emerge when these two principles come into conflict. Which one should take precedence? Is there a recognized method for determining what to do when two accepted ethical principles clash? When is it acceptable to seek to escape between the horns of the dilemma? There is no general response to these questions, but specific answers are forthcoming when individual cases are subjected to an ethical analysis.

## CASES OF TREATMENT REFUSAL: ETHICAL ANALYSIS

The following cases represent a spectrum ranging from patients who are clearly capable of decision making to somewhat impaired patients to those with a fluctuating or uncertain capacity. Complicating factors include the need for ongoing, periodic treatments such as dialysis, whether the advanced age of the patient should be a reason to respect treatment refusal, and whether the stance taken by the patient's family should influence the response of physicians.

### Case 1
Mr. A., a 62-year-old Jehovah's Witness, was admitted to the hospital with severe abdominal pains and a history of recurrent gallbladder disease. He underwent a cholecystectomy. After surgery he developed multiple complications, with gastrointestinal bleeding. He was a clear candidate for a blood transfusion, but because he had stated that he

was a Jehovah's Witness and did not want a transfusion, the procedure was withheld.

As his mental status began to deteriorate as a result of his poor health, a psychiatric consultation was requested. A mental-status examination was performed, and the patient was found not to be able to make any decisions concerning his treatment. His next of kin—a daughter—was contacted. She said that she was aware of her father's wishes, and as a Jehovah's Witness herself, refused to agree to a transfusion for her father.

The psychiatrist presenting the case framed the ethical questions: What is the extent of the physician's responsibility in treating a Jehovah's Witness patient who has refused to accept a blood transfusion in a life-threatening situation in the following cases?

A. The patient is competent to make a treatment decision.
B. The patient is incompetent to make a treatment decision.
C. The patient's family refuses to allow a blood transfusion.
D. The patient's family will grant permission for a blood transfusion in opposition to the patient's previously stated refusal when competent.

In situation A, psychiatrists experience discomfort, which they may mistake for an ethical problem. But there is no genuine ethical dilemma. The discomfort stems from the fact that a patient is refusing a low-risk medical procedure and, as a result, has a high probability of dying. The felt obligation of the psychiatrist is to act in accordance with the principle of beneficence and strive to bring about the beneficial consequence of saving the patient's life.

From the perspective of the patient in this case, however, there is a different and overriding consequence of accepting a blood transfusion: being "cut off" from eternal salvation. Jehovah's Witnesses have a metaphysical belief concerning the consequences of accepting blood transfusions and thus place a different value on preserving mortal life than do people who do not share their religious beliefs. Since ensuring eternal salvation ranks higher than preserving life here on earth, Witnesses have a different value hierarchy than do physicians who urge that a transfusion be given. For the psychiatrist to seek to override the patient's refusal would entail violating the principle of respect for autonomy. Justice Cardozo's dictum that "every human being of adult years and sound mind has a right to determine what shall be done with his own body" governs situation A, a Jehovah's Witness evaluated as having a "sound mind."

In situation B, it must first be ascertained whether the patient made his wishes about transfusion known prior to his becoming incompetent. It is ethically unacceptable to wait until a competent patient deteriorates and then administer the transfusion on the grounds that the patient is no longer competent and the situation has become an emergency. Law and ethics concur in recognizing an extension of autonomy in the case of patients who, while still competent, had clearly expressed their wishes about treatment.

Situation C introduces a new element, which alters the ethical analysis. Family members are frequently asked to consent to medical treatments on behalf of their relatives. But may they refuse a treatment, especially one that is low risk and stands to restore the patient's health? Where there is no evidence of what the patient's own wishes would be, the principle of respect for autonomy is inapplicable. It is the autonomy of the patient that must be respected, not that of the patient's family. In such cases, the obligation of the physician is solely that of beneficence, to strive to bring about a balance of good consequences over bad. If it is not known whether a particular Jehovah's Witness would accept a transfusion in a life-threatening situation, physicians may not simply take the family's refusal as a substitute for that of the patient.

Situation D is complicated by the fact that the family is seeking to act on the side of life, whereas the patient had, while competent, expressed the wish not to have blood transfusions. Physicians and hospital administrators no doubt will worry about legal liability if they fail to transfuse and the patient expires from loss of blood. However, from an ethical point of view, the resolution of the problem depends on the recency and certainty of the patient's previously expressed wishes. If, as in situation B, the patient was competent upon entering the hospital, and at that time clearly and unequivocally expressed the wish to refuse all transfusions, then respect for autonomy is the governing principle. When a patient's own recently stated wishes about treatment can be known with a reasonable degree of certainty, the family has no greater standing in requesting that treatment be given than in requesting that treatment be withheld. Nevertheless, as a practical matter, fear of liability contaminates ethical decision making, and a risk manager or hospital attorney typically will either decide in favor of transfusion or seek a judicial ruling to eliminate legal risks.

Although cases involving Jehovah's Witnesses' refusal of treatment are seen regularly in general hospitals, they are not nearly as common as cases in which elderly patients with mild dementia or depressed patients refuse a medically recommended procedure. Such cases pose genuine ethical dilemmas because of a large gray area in competency evaluations. Elderly patients often have fluctuating mental capacity, or they may consent to a treatment at one point and then later refuse the same treatment. Depressed patients can have a cognitive understanding of the purpose of a treatment, the procedures to be done, and the risks and benefits, and yet, owing to their mood disorder, they may refuse it. For example, they may take the risks of a treatment to be the benefits, as in the case of a depressed woman who, when told that the risks of dying from electroconvulsive therapy (ECT) were 1 in 3000, replied: "I hope I am the one" (Roth et al., 1977).

## Case 2

Ms. B. was 81 years old when she was admitted to the hospital with severe abdominal pains. She had decreased renal function, and a mass was found in her bladder. The patient was advised of the need for cystoscopy, which she refused. A psychiatric consultation was requested, and this first assessment found her to be competent. When the treatment team changed, a second psychiatric consultation was called, and on this evaluation Ms. B. was reassessed as "incompetent." The patient asserted her belief that penicillin would cure her, and she continued to refuse to allow a cystoscopic examination. When a third psychiatric consultation was called, the note on the chart read: "Patient appears weak, responds to questions, sometimes with humor. She has some paranoid ideas. Is alert and oriented. Mild dementia. Requires assistance to manage at home."

Cases like Ms. B.'s pose a problem of uncertain competency, where the uncertainty is unlikely to resolve. Does the ethical obligation require physicians to respect the patient's autonomy, or to strive to bring about the best medical outcome, based on their assessment of the patient's diminished autonomy? Ideally, a psychiatrist could succeed in persuading the recalcitrant patient to accept the treatment. Although it is coercive to force a patient to accept an unwanted treatment, an attempt at rational persuasion should not be viewed as coercive. To try to convince a resistant patient to accept a medical recommendation is to respect that patient's autonomy, not to violate it. However, if a physician's attempt to persuade involves threats of some kind, then an element of coercion has crept into the process. Attempts at rational persuasion do not always succeed, but time spent talking to patients often helps to establish a physician–patient relationship and gains the patient's trust.

There is no simple formula for determining when it is ethically permissible to override a patient's refusal of treatment on the basis of an assessment of diminished autonomy. In general, the more impaired the patient's thinking processes, the more acceptable it is to act in accordance with the principle of beneficence. An additional factor is the severity of the patient's medical condition and the consequences of not undertaking the therapy. The graver the consequences, the more acceptable it may be to override a marginally competent patient's refusal.

Opinion differs sharply on the relevance of the patient's age. Some argue explicitly that advanced age should be a reason to respect treatment refusals by patients with questionable competence because the use of expensive medical resources cannot be justified for people who have lived out what is considered to be their natural life span. Others adhere to the (often unwarranted) presumption that advanced age itself impairs thinking, and so paternalism can be justified. Both views are flawed from an ethical point of view. The first view introduces policy considerations into decision making at the bedside, which violates a principle of justice, and the second view ignores the obvious need to make clinical assessments in each individual case.

## THE "HARM" PRINCIPLE: BEYOND
## RESPECT FOR AUTONOMY

Situations in which patients refuse medical treatment or are judged to be dangerous to themselves test the limits of the principle of respect for autonomy. When physicians seek to override a patient's refusal of treatment or attempt to leave the hospital against medical advice, they are acting paternalistically: interfering with the patient's liberty for the patient's own good or welfare. Paternalistic behavior on the part of psychiatrists can be justified when patients lack full autonomy, although debates and uncertainty surround the precise circumstances in which such paternalism is ethically permissible.

A separate and distinct ethical principle comes into play when patients are judged dangerous to others. This principle, known as the harm principle, can be stated as follows: Interference with an individual's freedom or liberty of action can be justified when there is a reasonable likelihood that the person will cause harm to others. In the psychiatric context, the notion of harm to others is often lumped together with the notion of harm to self, as when a patient is evaluated as being "a danger to self or others." From an ethical point of view, however, the justification for interfering with a person's liberty or autonomy in these two situations rests on different principles. While it is paternalistic to interfere with a person's decisions or actions because of possible harm to self, it is not paternalistic to interfere with an individual's liberty or autonomy when that person is judged dangerous to others. In that circumstance, the justification is based on the harm principle.

The basis for the harm principle is usually taken to be the statement of the 19th-century British philosopher John Stuart Mill (1859/1961): "The only purpose for which power can be rightfully exercised over any member of a civilized community, against his will, is to prevent harm to others" (p. 263). Mill's version of the harm principle is explicitly antipaternalist. In his essay, he goes on to say: "[An individual's] own good, either physical or moral, is not a sufficient warrant. He cannot rightfully be compelled to do or forebear because it will be better for him to do so, because it will make him happier, because, in the opinions of others, to do so would be wise, or even right" (p. 263). Mill was writing about the relationship between the state and its citizens. He did not address the subject of psychiatric patients or other individuals who can be characterized as having diminished autonomy or as being legally incompetent.

Psychiatrists working in a general hospital are regularly confronted with situations that involve the need to evaluate patients who are potentially harmful to others, and to balance competing rights and interests in applying the harm principle.

## The Harm Principle and Confidentiality*

The respect-for-autonomy principle is typically associated with informed consent and decision making by patients, and yet it has other applications. Respect for autonomy is one variation of a broader principle known as respect for persons (National Commission for the Protection of Human Subjects, 1979). Dilemmas relating to privacy and confidentiality are additional areas in which the moral and legal rights of individuals are pitted against competing ethical concerns. The following two cases illustrate the complexity and interplay of several ethical principles. The resolution of these dilemmas is further complicated by laws and regulations whose applicability is uncertain.

## Case 3

Ms. C. was a 22-year-old sporadic intravenous drug user admitted to the psychiatric ward of a general hospital with a diagnosis of bipolar disorder. She had been living with her grandmother, with whom she had been having increasing verbal altercations. She agreed to voluntary admission when the emergency room psychiatrist evaluated her as out of control and in need of intensive inpatient treatment.

Even after medication was administered in the hospital, however, she remained out of control. Added to the difficulty of stabilizing this patient was a new problem that came to the attention of the staff on the inpatient psychiatric unit. The hospital is a large, inner city facility with typical staffing shortages. Adequate supervision is not available for all patients on the psychiatric ward, and it is known to the staff that patients have sexual intercourse with one another. It was discovered that Ms. C. had had sex with more than one of the patients on the ward. The staff members were uncertain about where their primary obligation lay and what course of action would be ethically permitted or required.

---

* The following sections of this article that relate to human-immunodeficiency-virus–positive psychiatric patients are adapted from a previously published article by this author (Macklin, 1991).

This situation is ethically problematic even without introducing the possibility of HIV infection. But in an era of the acquired immune deficiency syndrome (AIDS), with an estimated 50% to 60% of intravenous drug users in inner city areas testing positive for the HIV antibody, the risks of harm escalate. Added to the usual concerns about patients on hospital wards having sex with one another is the risk of transmitting the AIDS virus. Should Ms. C. be asked to undergo a blood test for HIV infection? Is it ethically or legally permissible to test her without her knowledge or consent? And what if she tests positive? What is the obligation to preserve confidentiality, and how should that obligation be weighed against the obligation to protect other patients?

When the case of Ms. C. was described at an ethics conference, different possible scenarios were sketched, each one giving rise to a different set of ethical problems. Consider the variations posed by the facts and circumstances. In variation 1, Ms. C. is offered a blood test for HIV infection and she refuses. In variation 2, she consents to the test. In variation 3, the patient responds to psychotropic medication and is ready for discharge, presumably back to the group home. In variation 4, she remains out of control and the decision is made to keep her on the psychiatric unit. Each scenario leads to a different, yet related set of ethical dilemmas of confidentiality and decisions about discharge, placement, and notification of persons who might be presumed to have a "need to know" that Ms. C. is HIV positive.

## Case 4

Mr. D. was a 42-year-old white male who was brought to the emergency room in an elated and grandiose state. After he was admitted to the inpatient unit, it became known that he had a long history of intravenous drug use and that he was HIV positive.

During his hospitalization, Mr. D. and Ms. E., another patient in the unit, developed a romantic relationship. They were seen close together during the day and at night. After Mr. D. was discharged, Ms. E. became hysterical, screaming, tearful, and extremely anxious. When approached by staff members, she stated that she had been having sex with Mr. D., and had been informed by one of the staff members that he had AIDS. She was medicated and placed on constant observation to prevent possible harm to self.

In contrast to the case of Ms. C., in this case, the physicians and staff knew that a patient on the inpatient unit was HIV positive. Furthermore, it was evident soon after his admission to the unit that he was involved romantically with another patient. It was never brought to the attention of the primary physician that the two patients were engaging in sexual activities, yet that possibility is always entertained even when patients are not romantically involved.

The psychiatrist who brought this case to the ethics conference summed up the ethical dilemma in these words: "How far can we go to protect third persons against a disease that might be lethal versus the patient's right to have privileged communication with the therapist?" Recast in the language of conflicting obligations, which of two legitimate obligations should take precedence: the obligation to preserve therapist–patient confidentiality or the obligation to take steps to prevent harm to others?

Even if the latter obligation is found to be primary, an ethical question can be raised about the action of the staff member who disclosed the confidential information to Ms. E. The timing and manner of such disclosures are important from an ethical point of view. To announce to a person that she has been placed at risk of acquiring a lethal infection, without providing adequate counseling and psychological support, exposes the patient to psychological harm in addition to the potential harm of HIV infection. When the individual is a psychiatric patient, the risk of harm may be substantially increased.

Both cases pose a question about the proper scope and limits of confidentiality. Yet the ethical issues go beyond confidentiality. In a period marked by AIDS, what precautions can be justified to prevent the transmission of HIV infection in an inpatient setting? Which means of exercising vigilance in monitoring patients' behavior are most acceptable? Is the isolation of patients known to be HIV positive ethically or legally permissible? Should mental health professionals adopt different standards regarding the discharge of HIV-infected psychiatric patients from those typically used for other psychiatric patients?

Since the AIDS epidemic began, two public-policy concerns have often come into conflict. The need to protect the health of uninfected people has led to proposals that endanger the civil liberties of persons with AIDS or HIV infection. An ethical analysis of the conflicting obligations surrounding HIV-infected psychiatric patients and confidentiality, as well as the issues that go beyond confidentiality, yields no simple answers. But the analysis can serve to clarify a complex of ethical, legal, and professional concerns by exposing some unquestioned assumptions and exploring analogies to related ethical problems in the mental health arena.

**Sex on the Hospital Wards**

Sexual contact between patients is generally prohibited on inpatient psychiatric units (Zonana, Norko, & Steir, 1988). From an ethical point of view, the underlying assumption appears to be that sex on the wards is not in the best interests of psychiatric patients. However, the basis for that position is not always clearly stated. At least the following three reasons might be invoked to support the prohibition:

1. A moralistic stance, for example, that sex among casual acquaintances is wrong and ought not be allowed in a health facility.
2. A legalistic worry. Hospital staff and administration fear potential liability if a patient feels wronged or harmed by a sexual encounter and brings a lawsuit against the hospital.
3. A principled ethical concern. Patients are vulnerable, whether they are physically or mentally ill, and a hospital has an obligation to protect them from exploitation and harm. Among the potential harms cited are risk of pregnancy, risk of venereal disease, and the possible harmful effect on the patient's condition that prompted hospitalization in the first place (Zonana et al., 1988).

Perhaps all three motives are at work, and there may be additional grounds for holding that sex between patients should be disallowed. But it is important to distinguish ethical justifications from other reasons. The only one of the three stated reasons that properly counts as an ethical basis for the prohibition is the third—that vulnerable people stand in need of protection against harm or exploitation, and an institution in which vulnerable people are housed has an obligation to take appropriate steps to ensure such protection. This ethical statement appears to be relatively uncontroversial, although disagreements are bound to arise about just how it is to be applied and when legitimate exceptions can be countenanced.

For ease of reference, let us term this statement the "vulnerability principle." One part of the vulnerability principle is based on the harm principle, which permits interference with individual liberty. The second part places an obligation on the institution, namely, to take appropriate steps to ensure the protection of vulnerable people housed there. Determining just which steps are appropriate also involves a value judgment, with practical constraints as well as ethical uncertainty.

Unlike the harm principle, the vulnerability principle is not narrowly antipaternalist. It permits interference with a *vulnerable* person's liberty for the purpose of preventing harm from befalling that person. The vulnerability principle would thus allow for a range of acts of ethically justified paternalism, restrictions on the behavior of vulnerable individuals to protect them from harm.

Zonana et al. (1988) note that "within many of the larger facilities, it is not possible to monitor sexual behavior without introducing draconian procedures, which would probably be ineffective and would undermine the therapeutic milieu" (p. 591). The ineffectiveness of such procedures alone would be sufficient argument against their use, from both an ethical and a practical standpoint. When the prospect of invasion of privacy and imposition of coercive measures is added, vigilant monitoring of the sexual behavior of inpatients becomes ethically unacceptable.

Legal constraints that limit what can be done to psychiatric patients have been put in place over the past few decades in response to earlier abuses. Judicial decisions and state regulations have established patients' rights to treatment, protecting them against indefinite "warehousing," as well as recognizing their right to refuse treatment, including psychotropic medication that could relieve symptoms. Most germane to the issue of controlling sexual behavior in the inpatient psychiatric setting, a general mandate exists to employ the "least restrictive alternative." That mandate would tend to render it legally impermissible to put patients in isolation. Appelbaum (1988) observes that control of sexual behavior in the hospital is problematic: "Isolation or seclusion in these cases will often seem inappropriate or may be precluded by state regulations" (p. 14).

If mental health staff members are typically distressed when they discover that patients on the psychiatric ward are having sex, they suffer even greater consternation when they suspect or learn that one of these patients is HIV positive. But short of placing patients in physical restraints or in isolation, the staff normally is powerless to halt these activities.

Despite legal prohibitions against unduly restrictive measures, the question of their ethical acceptability can be posed. Laws are sometimes changed for moral reasons, so it is always appropriate to ask whether current laws are too permissive or too stringent. The question of whether isolation of HIV-positive patients can be ethically justifiable can be answered by an appeal to the harm principle. However, the harm principle cannot stand alone as a basis for justification; it must be buttressed by relevant facts and probabilities regarding the magnitude and likelihood of harm.

The probability that harm is likely to befall patients in most situations would be too low to warrant isolation as an ethically acceptable strategy. This conclusion is based on an analogy with assessments of "dangerousness to others." Before a psychiatric patient deemed dangerous to others can be isolated, there must be a demonstrable likelihood of harm, as judged by competent professionals. The likelihood and magnitude of danger to others from HIV-infected patients should be evaluated according to analogous standards. Efforts should focus on those patients known by virtue of past behavior or current threats to represent a danger (Zonana et al., 1988).

Since it is risky behavior and not HIV positivity alone that transmits AIDS, the following conditions must be met before the isolation of an HIV-positive patient can be ethically considered: (1) the patient must be known to be, not merely suspected of being, HIV positive; (2) there must be solid evidence of the patient's propensity to engage in sexual behavior on the wards; and (3) the patient's inability or unwillingness to comply with safe sexual practices must be documented. Fulfillment of these three conditions does not render isolation ethically mandatory, but it does make it ethically permissible.

Condition 1 creates another problem, however. Recall the case of Ms. C. (Case 3). If a patient is not known to be seropositive, but as a documented intravenous drug user has a 50% to 60% chance of testing positive for the AIDS antibody, is it ethically or legally permissible to do a blood test for HIV infection? Legal constraints appear in state statutes, which vary throughout the nation. Many states have enacted laws that protect the rights of individuals not to be tested without their knowledge and consent.

## Problems of Confidentiality and Disclosure

In situations in which a patient is known to be HIV positive, as in the case of Mr. D. (Case 4), the ethical issues focus on confidentiality and disclosure. Since disclosure without permission constitutes a breach of confidentiality, the question is whether the objective of enabling other inpatients to protect themselves can justify the disclosure. This issue is complicated by the uncertainties surrounding the acquisition of HIV infection. Patients who have been exposed might already have become infected, and that could not be ascertained without doing a blood test for the antibody. However, since it can take up to six months, and possibly longer, for a person to develop antibodies to the AIDS virus, a negative test is not conclusive. These complexities suggest that only limited circumstances exist in which breach of confidentiality can be justified, when the basis for disclosing information is to enable other patients to protect themselves.

Couched in the most general terms, the ethical question is: When, if ever, may patient confidentiality be breached? As is true of almost all ethical questions, there is no right answer in the form of a moral absolute. Although an ethical absolutist might answer "Never!" the more common range of answers falls along a continuum from "very rarely" to "when the situation warrants it." More important than a statistical reckoning of what physicians in general, mental health professionals in particular, or members of the public think about this issue is the reasons they give. In examining the ethics of breaching confidentiality, it is necessary to see whether those reasons stand up to moral scrutiny.

In a therapeutic setting, there is a strong presumption in favor of preserving confidentiality of information that relates to patients' and clients' diagnoses, prognoses, and other facts. The reasons for having ethical principles and laws protecting therapist–patient confidentiality are several. First, clinical information is intensely private, and disclosure to unauthorized persons has the potential for harming a patient's interests. There is ample evidence to support the view that the interests of people with AIDS have been seriously harmed by disclosure of their HIV infection: the loss of housing, of jobs, and of insurance are among the documented consequences for many individuals.

Second, the therapist–client relationship is built on trust. When physicians breach confidentiality, they undermine trust, damage the physician–patient relationship, and possibly interfere with the therapeutic process. This last factor is especially important in the mental health context, which is why confidentiality in the therapist–patient relationship is held to be especially important.

The most frequently cited legal precedent in the mental health arena is the "duty to warn," established in the *Tarasoff* case decided in California in 1976. Although the *Tarasoff* case involved a psychiatric patient, setting a precedent for the obligation of therapists to do something to protect specific persons from being harmed by an individual whom they judge to be violent or dangerous, the court in *Tarasoff* "based its decision in part on its reading of earlier cases holding physicians liable for failing to inform family members of the infectious nature of a patient's condition" (Appelbaum, 1988, p. 14). The original precedents, then, for situations of presumed dangerousness to others are those of persons with infectious diseases rather than of persons considered likely to harm others by violent behavior.

The principal reason for allowable breach centers on harm to others that might result if confidentiality is not breached. But this only invites a series of subsidiary questions: How high should the probability be that such harm will occur? On what is the assessment of probability based? Do experts agree on that assessment? How serious must the probable harm be? Are there alternative means for seeking to prevent it besides breaching confidentiality? To whom may disclosure be made? To authorities, such as the police? To other health-care professionals or administrators? To the patient's family? To an employer? Must the patient be informed that the physician intends to disclose confidential information? If so, must the patient be informed prior to disclosure? Or is it sufficient to notify the patient after the disclosure has been made? Will disclosure of confidential information actually have the intended effect, whatever that effect is? Answers to these questions are neither clear nor simple.

## Confidentiality and AIDS

Eth (1988) finds it ironic "that while psychiatrists were initially reluctant to accept the *Tarasoff* doctrine, physicians are now in the vanguard of extending this duty to protect the sexual partners of HIV-infected patients . . . " (p. 576).

Guidelines set forth by a number of professional organizations have addressed the issue of disclosure of a patient's HIV status to a spouse or other known regular sex partners. For example, the AIDS Policy Statement issued by the American Psychiatric Association permits confidentiality to be breached when an HIV-positive patient continues to engage in high-risk behavior: "It is ethically permissible for the physician to notify an identifiable person who the physician believes is in danger of contracting the virus" (Eth, 1988, p. 571).

Statements about what is ethically permissible provide only weak guidance, however. Ethical duties and obligations embrace three categories: (1) that which is ethically obligatory, (2) that which is ethically prohibited, and (3) that which is ethically permissible. Of the three, the third allows for the widest discretion on the part of moral agents. Health professionals seeking moral guidance from statements of professional organizations or from the law will probably be disappointed with this lack of precision. The psychiatric AIDS policy statement is explicit in absolving psychiatrists of an absolute obligation to preserve confidentiality. In so doing, it creates ethical ambiguity.

A reliance on the "duty to warn" presupposes that issuing a verbal warning to patients at risk would be sufficient to protect them. Yet some psychiatric patients may fail to comprehend the warning, others may choose not to act appropriately even given the warning, and others may actually experience a worsening of their psychiatric disorder.

This last possibility is noted by one psychiatrist who surmises that informing a paranoid schizophrenic patient that he or she might have contracted a fatal disease—despite the minuscule probability (the patient bit another patient who was HIV positive on the cheek, drawing blood)—would have made him or her extremely anxious and might have worsened his or her psychiatric condition (Binder, 1987).

Although not all psychiatric patients have impaired cognition, those who are impaired may be unable to understand the nature and consequences of their HIV infection, their actions, or both. This group would presumably lack the understanding that is a prerequisite for refraining from transmitting the HIV virus to others. Breach of confidentiality might then be justified on the grounds that these individuals lack the mental capacity to prevent harm to others.

Similarly, although not all psychiatric patients lack the ability to control their behavior, some do exhibit behavior that is out of control. Despite the fact that an HIV-infected individual may have a cognitive understanding of the nature and consequences of his or her behavior, the risks of spreading the infection remain.

Then there are those individuals in whom the two impairments are combined, a situation thought to exist in a considerable number of HIV-infected patients—those with dementia or AIDS encephalopathy. "This organic brain syndrome is associated with progressive mental deterioration and disintegration in cognition, emotion, and behavior. It may occasion changes in behavior patterns such as disinhibited sexual activity, aggressiveness, and loss of self-care skills" (Gostin, 1987, p. 64). The significant incidence of AIDS encephalopathy thus blurs the distinction between HIV-infected individuals who are not psychiatric patients and psychiatric patients who have HIV infection. Many in the first group will become members of the second by virtue of the effect of AIDS on their brains.

A distinctly different problem is what to do about those who are unwilling to change or control their behavior, a characteristic of individuals who may not be diagnosed as having a mental disorder, but rather are labeled as having antisocial personality disorder. These people cannot truly be called mentally incompetent, yet the risk they pose to others may be as great as or greater than that of psychiatric patients.

For individuals who fall within any of these groups, the harm principle can justify suspending the usual confidentiality mandate that protects other HIV-infected individuals. However, this conclusion cannot be based simply on the psychiatric diagnosis. Instead, it must be based on evidence supporting the likelihood that they will engage in behavior that will place others at risk.

An unjustified breach of confidentiality was described in a case referred to above:

> [This was a] case of a 22-year-old heterosexual, married man with a diagnosis of paranoid schizophrenia. While being evaluated for management of agitation and increased delusional ideas, he suddenly ran out of the interview room, which is located on the unit, and bit another patient on the cheek, drawing blood. The bitten patient had had a positive AIDS antibody result.

> The question was raised as to whether we should tell the paranoid schizophrenic patient that he had come in contact with a small amount of the blood of a patient with positive AIDS antibody. On the one hand, did he not have the right to know that he might have contracted a fatal disease? On the other hand, . . . the likelihood of the patient's contracting AIDS was minimal. (Binder, 1987, p. 179)

This is an example of a false dilemma that stems from flawed ethical reasoning. The reasoning is flawed because of the minuscule possibility of becoming infected from one bite on the cheek of an infected person. Unless the one doing the biting is Count Dracula, there is little to suggest that the amount of blood drawn and the probability of its entering the biter's bloodstream could produce AIDS (Friedland & Klein, 1987). In order to justify a departure from the usual dictates of confidentiality, the consequences of not breaching confidentiality must be of considerable magnitude and reasonably likely to occur. The case of the cheek bite fails to suggest any such consequences. Indeed, the author of the case cites only one potential negative consequence of telling the patient who did the biting: "This knowledge would have made him extremely anxious and might have worsened his psychiatric condition" (Binder, 1987, p. 179).

To reach an ethically acceptable conclusion that breach of confidentiality is justified, it is not enough to ask what circumstances might warrant disclosure of a psychiatric patient's HIV status. It must also be determined what is to be done following the disclosure of that information. One possibility pertains to disclosure regarding patients about to be released—disclosure to family or to care givers at a subsequent institution. This dilemma confronted the staff in the case of Ms. C. once the patient consented to an HIV test and was found to be seropositive. Even when there is a law that permits disclosure on a "need to know" basis, professionals should seek to maintain confidentiality protections.

There may be good reasons for personnel at a nursing home to be aware that some residents may be HIV positive. This would enable the staff to mount an educational program within the home, to institute universal precautions recommended for handling blood and other bodily fluids, and to look out for any manifest signs of disease in residents so they might be referred for medical treatment. However, information about an individual's HIV status cannot be used as a reason for refusal to admit that person into the home. Such a refusal would violate ethical and legal prohibitions against discrimination.

A more troubling dilemma, beyond confidentiality, could stem from the judgment that a psychiatric patient is too "dangerous" to be released either to home or to another institutional setting. This would be, in effect, a decision to confine the patient indefinitely, to isolate an HIV-infected person on the grounds of dangerousness to others.

The ethical basis for rejecting involuntary commitment as a general strategy is the familiar and compelling civil libertarian position that the only legitimate ground for incarceration is the actual commission of a crime. Anything else amounts to preventive detention, a practice that is anathema in a free society. This position is often buttressed by the minority opinion issued in the *Tarasoff* case: predictions of dangerousness are too unreliable to allow them to be used as grounds for incarcerating someone. According to a view at one extreme of the civil libertarian spectrum, even if much more accurate predictions were possible, it would still be unacceptable to incarcerate persons in advance of their having committed a criminal act.

A contrasting view holds that if accurate predictions of future behavior could be made, then preventive detention could be ethically justified. As Zonana et al. (1988) argue:

Civil commitment may be an appropriate response to the mentally ill patient who poses a danger to others by engaging in behaviors with a high risk of HIV transmission . . . . Just as an acutely psychotic patient who expressed homicidal ideation and possessed a weapon would be involuntarily committed, so might a psychotic patient known to be HIV positive who expressed a desire to spread the disease to others via sexual contact or shared needles. The physician must clearly understand, however, that the basis for commitment is not the patient's HIV status or sexual behavior, but the patient's mental illness that creates danger to others. (pp. 591–592)

Numerous situations are bound to arise in which a mental health professional is confronted by a choice between, on the one hand, preserving confidentiality and isolating the patient, and, on the other, disclosing the patient's HIV infection to individuals who might be placed at risk or who will be in charge of the patient's care. Given this choice, the ethical priority is clear. It is less restrictive, and therefore ethically preferable, to breach confidentiality than to take away a person's liberty by confining him or her indefinitely.

The obligation of clinicians in an inpatient setting may well be increased by the fact that the persons at risk are other hospital patients to whom the care givers owe a duty to provide a safe, therapeutic environment. Nevertheless, it remains unclear how that duty is to be fulfilled.

## FAMILY PROBLEMS AND ADMINISTRATIVE DECISIONS

From a practical standpoint, insurmountable barriers often confront psychiatrists who seek to make ethically sound decisions and to act in accordance with them. Two commonly encountered barriers are the families of psychiatric patients and hospital or nursing home administrators. The following cases are illustrative.

### Case 5

Mr. F., a 52-year-old man with a long history of psychiatric illness, was brought to the psychiatric emergency room of the general hospital by his wife because he had been drinking, talking loudly and irrelevantly, and threatening his family and passersby. He was admitted on an emergency status and started on his regular medication. He complied well with treatment and responded quickly. After three weeks of hospitalization, the treatment team agreed that he had reached his baseline functioning and was ready for discharge. His wife was informed, and follow-up was appropriately arranged. He agreed with the plans and was looking forward to going home.

On the morning of the discharge day, his social worker in the inpatient unit received a call from the patient's wife, who said that Mr. F. was not ready for discharge. An hour later, the psychiatrist received another phone call, from an unidentified woman, stating that Mr. F. was "crazy" and that discharge was not appropriate at this time. The situation was discussed at team rounds and the patient was interviewed. He was considered not to be a danger to self or others and was deemed appropriate for discharge. The team decided to discharge him that day, although the situation at home was not clear and there was a high probability that the patient would be brought back to the hospital by the family. In fact, the family did bring him back that same day.

The dilemma, as stated by the psychiatrist, was as follows: To what extent should the treatment team members use their power to retain a patient whom they know will be going to an environment that will promote immediate decompensation and necessitate readmission? How does the ethical psychiatrist protect a patient from being forced back into the hospital by family or friends without violating the patient's rights and welfare? Unlike ethical dilemmas that arise out of a conflict between ethical principles, this type of ethical problem stems from the actions of people outside the therapist–patient relationship. When those "outsiders" are the patient's own family, there is little the psychiatrist can do to advocate further for the patient. However, when outsiders are other actors in the health-care system, it calls for some reform within the system itself, as the next case demonstrates.

## Case 6

Ms. G. was a 67-year-old woman referred directly to the hospital admissions office by her nursing home because she was not following "home rules." The administrator contacted the emergency room and requested a medical/psychiatric evaluation of the patient. From Ms.

G.'s old chart, it was learned that she was suffering from Alzheimer-type dementia and recently had been discharged from the medical service at the acute-care hospital after six months of continual hospitalization. The reason that Ms. G. had remained in the hospital so long was that she had become a "disposition problem"; her family refused to take her back and social workers were unable to arrange another placement.

The hospital administrator contacted the psychiatric resident who had evaluated Ms. G. and told the resident to "try not to admit the patient" because of the potential disposition problem. The nursing home was contacted and informed that the patient did not meet the criteria for admission to the psychiatric unit. However, the nurse in charge at the nursing home refused to accept Ms. G. back on the grounds that her staff was unable to manage her. While negotiations were going on between the hospital and nursing home administrator, Ms. G. wandered out of the hospital.

The sad case of Ms. G. demonstrates how patients can be both harmed and wronged by the actions of administrators, whose concerns are often at odds with the interests of patients. It also shows how the ability of doctors to advocate for their patients is diminishing as hospital administrators wield greater power. The nursing home was seeking to "dump" a patient who had become a "management problem," and used as a justification the patient's violation of the nursing home's rules. The hospital administrator desperately tried not to readmit the patient in order to avoid a predictable repetition of the "disposition problem" this patient had already posed. The psychiatric resident tried to comply with the hospital administrator's recommendation by invoking a medically respectable justification: the patient did not fit the criteria for admission to the acute-care psychiatric ward. There was no one left with the power or authority to advocate for the unfortunate Ms. G.

Although the ethical principle applicable to this case is quite clear, and there is no conflict of principles to create an ethical dilemma, the barriers to a mental health professional who sought to act in his patient's best interest were formidable. The psychiatrist had no recourse in the face of decisions by administrators at two different facilities, administrators who appeared to have ultimate authority to act, but lacked an ethical basis for their decisions.

## CONCLUSION

The issues discussed in this chapter are representative of ethical dilemmas and problems that confront psychiatrists in the general hospital. The attempt was not to present an exhaustive listing of ethical issues, but, to provide sample cases, accompanied by an ethical analysis, in order to depict the sources of ethical problems, their complexity, and the principles that can be used in trying to resolve them.

The reasons why it is often impossible to arrive at a definitive or uncontroversial resolution of an ethical problem should now be clearer. Patients who have both a medical disease and a psychiatric illness present complex problems, with ethical, legal, and psychosocial dimensions. A patient's fluctuating or uncertain competency creates doubts about the degree to which autonomy should be respected and whether autonomy has become so diminished that decisions should no longer be left to the patient. Conflicts between adhering to the principle of beneficence and to the principle of respect for autonomy may leave a psychiatrist torn between these competing values. Moreover, reasonable people disagree about which principle should take precedence on the occasions when they conflict.

Uncertainty surrounding the probability that a patient will do harm to others, or about the magnitude of such potential harm, creates the dilemma of choosing between conflicting obligations: to preserve the patient's liberty and confidentiality or to act to prevent possible harm to others. In the present era of AIDS, the traditional problem of patients judged dangerous to others because of their propensity for violence is broadened to include HIV-infected psychiatric patients who lack the understanding or the control to refrain from risking the spread of the lethal disease. These are only some of the numerous and varied ethical concerns that arise in the general hospital.

Additional situations are those in which ethical problems stem not from a conflict of principles or from uncertainty regarding facts or probabilities, but from actions by hospital and nursing home administrators or the behavior of members of patients' families. There may be little psychiatrists can do to alter rejection of or hostility to patients by members of their families. But it is to be hoped that both individual psychiatrists and the profession as a whole will challenge the authority and power of administrators whose decisions and actions violate patients' rights, override their autonomy, and cause harm to their interests.

## REFERENCES

Appelbaum, P. S. (1988). AIDS, psychiatry, and the law. *Hospital and Community Psychiatry, 139,* 13–14.

Beauchamp, T. L., & Childress, J. F. (1989). *Principles of biomedical ethics* (3d ed.). New York: Oxford University Press.

Binder, R. L. (1987). AIDS antibody tests on inpatient psychiatry units. *American Journal of Psychiatry, 144,* 176–181.

Eth, S. (1988). The sexually active, HIV infected patient: Confidentiality versus the duty to protect. *Psychiatric Annals, 18,* 571–576.

Friedland, G., & Klein, R. (1987). Transmission of the human immunodeficiency virus. *New England Journal of Medicine, 317,* 1125–1135.

Gostin, L. (1987). Traditional public health strategies. In H. L. Dalton, S. Burris, & the Yale AIDS Law Project (Eds.), *AIDS and the law* (pp. 47–65). New Haven, CT: Yale University Press.

Macklin, R. (1991). HIV-infected psychiatric patients: Beyond confidentiality. *Ethics and Behavior, I,* 3–20.

Mill, J. S. (1961). On liberty. In M. Lerner (Ed.), *Essential works of John Stuart Mill* (pp. 254–360). New York: Bantam. (Original work published 1859.)

National Commission for the Protection of Human Subjects of Biomedical and Behavioral Research (1979). *The Belmont report: Ethical principles and guidelines for the protection of human subjects of research.* Washington, DC: Department of Health, Education, and Welfare.

Roth, L. H., Meisel, A., & Lidz, C. W. (1977). Tests of competency to consent to treatment. *American Journal of Psychiatry, 134,* 279–284.

*Schloendorff v. New York Hospital,* 211 N.Y. 129, 105 NE 92 (1914).

Zonana, H., Norko, M., & Steir, D. (1988). The AIDS patient on the psychiatric unit: Ethical and legal issues. *Psychiatric Annals, 18,* 587–593.

# PART II
# Psychiatric Emergency and Inpatient Services

3

# Emergency Room Psychiatric Care in the General Hospital
## Major Psychiatric–Legal Considerations

SHELDON TRAVIN

Clinicians practicing in general hospital emergency rooms need to become more aware of basic legal issues relevant to decision making in the assessment and management of psychiatric patients. In recent years, more and more psychiatric patients have been coming to emergency rooms for help; at the same time, the legal regulations concerning psychiatric practice have expanded significantly. Because the majority of general hospitals do not have psychiatrists and other mental health professionals stationed in their emergency rooms, clinicians covering the emergency services are required, at least initially, to assess and manage psychiatric patients coming there. As in all hospital emergency room care, physicians should adhere to the rule of reasonable care, and should personally examine the patients. Moreover, clinicians should bear in mind that the decisions they make concerning psychiatric patients frequently involve the resolution of complex psychiatric–legal issues.

A number of factors have converged to account for the increased utilization of hospital emergency rooms by psychiatric patients. These include the impetus given by the Community Mental Health Centers Act of 1963, which mandated that emergency psychiatric treatment be provided in federally funded community mental health centers; the phenomenon of deinstitutionalization that resulted in the use of emergency rooms by discharged state hospital patients for help with their chronic problems; and the disappearance of the general practitioner

51

from depressed areas, which further narrowed the already limited treatment resources for the urban poor (Bassuk & Gerson, 1979). As Linn (1971) has suggested, general hospital emergency room psychiatry has become "a gateway to community medicine."

In addition to the wide range of inherently complex psychiatric–legal issues that they routinely face with psychiatric patients in the emergency room, clinicians' difficulties are compounded by the atmosphere of marked uncertainty that is unavoidable given the frequent unavailability of sufficient relevant data and information, inadequate time to establish a therapeutic relationship, and a compelling need to make decisions rapidly. Appelbaum and Gutheil (1991) point out that because of the usual limitations of resources, particularly those of time and information, clinicians assessing patients in the emergency context cannot be held to the same standard of thoroughness as those expected in nonemergency situations. The key questions are two: Did the clinician make a reasonable attempt to obtain the necessary information? Given the circumstances, did the clinician perform in an adequate manner? Above all, the clinician cannot defer his or her decision making about the patient's emergency condition; indeed, the clinician may be held legally accountable if his or her indecisiveness results in harm to the patient. Tancredi (1982) emphasizes that in tense emergency situations, especially when limited information is available, clinicians tend to act in the most conservative way. Consequently, he cautions that these clinicians should be especially alert to considering patients' rights. The clinician must be sensitive to the accuracy of his or her evaluation and to the need to balance the competing interests of the patient's rights to autonomy and self-determination and the clinician's "therapeutic power" in deciding whether to commit a patient or treat the patient on an outpatient basis (Tancredi, 1982). Essentially, clinicians must consider the ethical and legal issues involving the rights of patients before they decide to restrict those prerogatives in any way (Tancredi, 1982).

## INITIATION OF EMERGENCY PSYCHIATRIC CARE

With its fundamental subjectivity, the definition of what constitutes a psychiatric emergency is more problematic than the usual definition of a medical emergency with its demonstrable physicality (Swartz, 1987). "Although readily observable dangerous behaviors (police power emergencies) may develop in a psychiatric emergency, there are inner emergent states such as imminent psychotic decompensations (*parens patriae* emergencies) that are recognized only by subtle clinical skills" (Swartz, 1987, p. 61). Whereas lack of consent in a medical emergency evokes the use of the emergency exception rule for treatment, refusal of treatment by a patient in a psychiatric emergency, which is a common occurrence, is a more complex issue. The tendency to rely on dangerousness rather than *parens patriae* as a justification for emergency intervention has complicated clinical discretion (Swartz, 1987).

Once a hospital has established an emergency room, a duty is created to treat patients who are in medical crises. Moreover, medicolegal authorities concur that only a physician has the necessary training to diagnose an emergency, except in an obviously life-threatening situation, when a nurse may declare an emergency. Generally speaking, a psychiatrist should declare a psychiatric emergency and render immediate treatment. However, if a psychiatrist is not available, then the physician on duty should initiate some form of intervention to stabilize the patient until the psychiatrist arrives to assume responsibility for the case. Halleck (1980) has emphasized that a physician assigned to the emergency room cannot refuse to see any patient who appears. The physician must consider every patient to be an emergency case until he or she personally examines the patient and determines otherwise. At the time the physician sees the patient, a physician–patient relationship is established. There now exists a duty of care, in addition to an ethical obligation to provide service, to find another doctor or suitable disposition, and to be available to the patient until this is satisfactorily accomplished. Julavits (1983) points out that the emergency psychiatric patient should not have to wait an unreasonable length of time before being seen by the psychiatrist for definitive treatment. Consequently, every effort should be made not to keep the patient waiting excessively. During this waiting period, emergency room personnel must take the precautions necessary to ensure the safety of both the patient and others. A failure to control and protect the patient awaiting treatment could constitute a breach of duty to the patient (Julavits, 1983).

## ORGANIC VERSUS FUNCTIONAL
## PSYCHIATRIC DISORDERS

In the emergency evaluation of a psychotic patient, Dubin and Weiss (1986) have noted that the most important clinical decision consists of "differentiating between organic mental disease (OMD) and functional psychiatric illness" (p. 147). Failure to make this crucial differentiation may delay appropriate treatment and could result in severe harm to the patient. Halleck (1980) has commented that, while the doctrine of negligent diagnosis has commonly been the basis for legal action in most medical specialties, this doctrine, for the most part, has been restricted as the cause of action in cases of suicide or harm to others in psychiatric practice. But with the expanding information on physical dysfunction producing or masquerading as psychological symptomatology, psychiatric clinicians will need to be concerned with the physical evaluation of the patient. The revised third edition of the *Diagnostic and Statistical Manual of Mental Disorders* (DSM-III-R) characterizes "organic mental disorder" as "a particular kind of organic mental syndrome in which the organic factor is known or presumed" and "may be a primary disease of the brain or a systemic illness that secondarily affects the brain. It may also be a psychoactive substance or toxic agent . . ." (American Psychiatric Association, 1987, p. 98).

Therefore, clinicians need to be cognizant of the fact that a significant number of patients presenting for emergency evaluation have psychiatric symptoms that are produced by unrecognized physical illness (Hall & Beresford, 1986). In a study of 658 consecutive psychiatric outpatients seen in initial evaluations, Hall and colleagues (Hall, Popkin, Devaul, Faillace, & Stickney, 1978) found that 9.1% of these patients had a medical condition believed to be the cause of the psychiatric symptoms. Of these patients identified with medically induced psychiatric disorders, 28% experienced visual hallucinations, distortions, or illusions. The most frequent medical conditions causing psychiatric symptoms were cardiovascular, endocrine, infectious, and pulmonary disorders. Johnson (1968) has argued that because physical illness is a major factor in precipitating psychiatric symptoms, a full physical examination should be performed to establish a reliable diagnosis.

Leeman (1975) points out, as well, that because many patients visiting general hospital emergency rooms present with mixed physical and psychological problems, it is extremely important that clinicians consider both aspects of a patient's illness. These mixed presentations include "physical complaints apparently due to psychological causes, injuries and illnesses secondary to psychological factors, psychological sequelae of illness or injury, and apparently unrelated physical and psychological problems occurring in the same patient" (Leeman, 1975, p. 533). Leeman cautions clinicians, therefore, not to come to hasty conclusions about patients on the basis of single facts that might lead to their problems' being labeled as either "psychiatric" or "organic." Moreover, the error of a premature diagnosis would be compounded by the psychiatrist's accepting conclusively, without any further consideration, that the patient was "medically cleared" by the nonpsychiatric physician (Weissberg, 1979). Weissberg maintains that the term "medically clear," though it sounds definitive, is actually ambiguous, and has been applied in potentially misleading ways, at times creating a false assurance and an impediment to the correct evaluation of the patient. He believes that the overuse of the term may be related to the nonpsychiatric physician's unfamiliarity or discomfort with clinical psychiatry and to the psychiatrist's overreliance on the medical opinion of nonpsychiatric physicians. He further believes that both of these shortcomings should be addressed in graduate medical education, with emphasis placed on the training and collaboration among the various specialties and on the physical integration of services. Melinek, Bluestone, and Steinmuller (1983) showed that the presence of a consulting psychiatrist at medical rounds in a city hospital emergency room had a positive impact on the medical staff members by raising their sensitivity to psychological topics.

## Case 1: Organic Mental Disorder

Mr. A., a 69-year-old widower with a long history of both recurrent major depression and chronic obstructive pulmonary disease (COPD), was brought, in a highly agitated state, by ambulance from an adult residence into the emergency room of a busy inner-city general hospital. A counselor from the residence who accompanied him reported that over the past 24 hours, the patient's behavior had changed dramatically. The counselor described Mr. A. as displaying erratic behavior, frequently alternating between marked restlessness and sluggishness. He had become very argumentative; he maintained that everybody was going to be killed, and on one occasion he pushed and slapped a staff member. He complained at times of seeing "lights" on the wall, and at other times, that he was being held captive in a police station or elsewhere; he seemed to be totally confused. What was remarkable was that the patient had been attending the mental health clinic regularly, and, until this sudden change, he seemed to be doing well. He had also been attending the medical clinic, where his condition was considered stable.

In the emergency room, Mr. A. was noted to be breathing rapidly, but he refused to allow the nurse to take his vital signs. Because the patient was agitated, belligerent, and threatening, and because he was known to be a "psychiatric patient," the triage nurse referred him to the psychiatric emergency service.

The psychiatrist who attempted to interview Mr. A. found him sitting in a wheelchair. His breathing was rapid, shallow, and somewhat painful, and he was restless and could not sit still. He was unable to maintain attention to the questions and switched subjects rapidly. He was disoriented as to time and place, with immediate and recent memory impairments, and his thinking was markedly disorganized. He verbalized paranoid fear that someone was going to kill him, and he misinterpreted the nurse's conversation outside the room as having some special reference to him. He denied wanting to kill himself or anyone else. Based on the counselor's report and his own interview, the psychiatrist presumptively diagnosed organic mental disorder, probably delirium secondary to an underlying medical condition, and referred the patient to the medical emergency service.

When the medical internist began the physical examination, the patient became severely agitated and combative. Although the internist's presumptive diagnosis was also delirium, he requested a specific psychiatric determination of the patient's capacity to give informed consent before he would initiate treatment against the patient's will. After again interviewing the patient, the psychiatrist wrote a detailed note on the chart explaining that the patient lacked the mental capacity to weigh the risk and benefits and to make a reasoned decision about the need for treatment. The medical internist then ordered restraints, as well as the intramuscular administration of a very small dose of Haldol (haloperidol) to calm him, after which he initiated a thorough medical examination. The patient's temperature was found to be 101°F, and a chest x-ray revealed an opacity in the left lower lobe of his lung. The clinical diagnosis was left lower lobe pneumonia.

*Discussion of Case 1*

Several medicolegal decisions were made in this case. Recognizing the organic nature of the presenting disorder, the psychiatrist immediately referred the patient to the medical service for consultation and specialty care. Because the patient had been reported as symptomatic for at least 24 hours, the medical internist believed the situation was urgent, but felt that he needed a determination of the patient's competency to give informed consent before he could initiate treatment against the patient's will. The presumption is always that the patient is competent until determined by examination to be otherwise. Once it has been determined that the patient lacks the mental capacity to make a decision as to treatment and is suffering from a health-deteriorating condition that is documented in the chart, medical treatment can be initiated. In general, the hospital's risk management is contacted and further legal action is considered.

With regard to the legal aspects of the management of delirium, Fogel, Mills, and Landen (1986) point out that in a true emergency situation, the common law doctrine of implied consent for treatment would apply. However, if the delirious patient requires urgent but not necessarily emergency medical treatment, the situation is more ambiguous legally. "The urgency of the clinical situation and the risk-to-benefit ratio of the proposed intervention will determine how extensive and formal such third party [for decision making] needs to be" (Fogel et al., 1986, p. 155). Although state statutes restrict the use of neuroleptic agents in functional mental disorders, Fogel and colleagues underscore that it is standard medical practice to use them for severely agitated or combative delirious patients. This amounts to an extension of the implied consent doctrine and enables the necessary diagnostic and therapeutic procedures to be performed. It would also be grossly inappropriate to apply civil commitment procedure to patients suffering from delirium whose organic etiology may be reversed with medical treatment (Fogel et al., 1986).

## PSYCHOACTIVE SUBSTANCE–INDUCED ORGANIC MENTAL DISORDER

In addition to organic mental disorders associated with physical disorders, clinicians should be aware of the problematic nature of psychoactive substance–induced organic mental disorders, as well as the extent of the cooccurrence of substance abuse disorders and mental disorders in patients coming to general hospital emergency rooms. In a study of 343 consecutive patients referred to a general hospital's emergency psychiatric service, Szuster, Schanbacher, and McCann (1990) found that 114 patients (33%) had an alcohol- and/or drug-induced disorder. Of these 114 patients, 68 (60%) were diagnosed as having either alcohol- or drug-induced disorders and 46 (40%) as having an alcohol- or drug-induced disorder concomitant with another mental disorder. These patients with alcohol- or drug-induced disorders were more likely to be male, young, unemployed, and homeless, as well as having increased frequencies of suicidal behavior. Importantly, alcohol was found to be the main substance contributing to psychiatric emergencies. In view of the consistent reports in the literature of the frequent cooccurrence of substance abuse disorders and mental disorders, Lehman, Meyers, and Corty (1989) emphasize that clinicians should thoroughly assess the possibility of dual diagnoses in their patients. Ananth et al. (1989) are concerned about what they believe to be a common failure to detect drug abuse or addiction in many psychotic patients seen in emergency rooms. These researchers emphasize that drug abuse or addiction is much more common than is generally diagnosed, and that drug usage markedly complicates the clinical presentation and management.

### Case 2: Alcohol Intoxication

Mr. B., a 41-year-old divorced, sporadically employed man who lived alone, came into the general hospital's emergency room in the early evening and requested alcohol detoxification because he was feeling "bad." He had been hospitalized previously on an alcohol detoxification unit in another hospital, but had never been hospitalized psychiatrically. Clearly under the influence of alcohol, Mr. B. had considerable difficulty concentrating, but was able to describe his having drunk heavily in the past several months because of depressive feelings after his girlfriend had left him.

During the psychiatric examination, the patient was found to have a flushed face, slurred speech, and a somewhat unsteady gait. His mood was severely depressed, and he acknowledged having thoughts that he would be better off dead and that from time to time he considered killing himself. He had occasionally heard his name being called, and once or twice he thought he saw "shadows." He was oriented as to place and person, but not to date. Insight and judgment were judged to be impaired. A breath analyzer test revealed moderate alcohol intoxication. Physical examination by the consulting medical internist showed no unusual findings.

Because there were no beds on the alcohol detoxification unit, the patient agreed to sleep overnight in an observation bed located in the psychiatric emergency service of the emergency room and to be re-evaluated in the morning. A blood sample was drawn for an alcohol-level test and a urine sample was obtained for toxicology screening.

The next morning, the patient was found to be alert and fully oriented, without any signs of inebriation. However, he remained severely depressed, and he admitted that he still had suicidal thoughts and would probably attempt to kill himself once outside. Upon further questioning, he admitted that he had planned to kill himself if he had been released from the hospital the night before. Moreover, he stated that he had been feeling severely depressed on and off for nearly two years, and had attempted suicide by hanging a year earlier after a quarrel with his girlfriend. However, he said that he was now feeling better physically, and that he wanted to sign himself out of the hospital to "take care of a number of things at home." Mr. B. flatly refused to consider voluntary admission to the psychiatric ward to be treated for his alcohol problem and severe depression. Having determined that the patient was a serious risk for suicide, the psychiatrist admitted him involuntarily to the psychiatric ward on an emergency basis. On the psychiatric ward, alcohol detoxification was started, and supplemented by treatment for depression.

*Discussion of Case 2*

The psychiatric–legal decisions pertaining to this case depend on an understanding both of the emergency care services for persons intoxicated with alcohol and of the commitment criteria for dangerous-to-self patients. Clinicians need to be aware that alcoholic patients requesting detoxification and help for their drinking problems are often sent to the hospital at the request of relatives, and that these relatives, as well as the patients themselves, may not be fully aware of the patients' other mental or medical problems. Even if the patient has some notion of such problems, he or she may minimize them and concentrate solely on the obvious drinking problem. Consequently, it is imperative that all detoxification patients be adequately screened prior to admission to the detoxification unit.

With regard to acutely intoxicated persons, most states have statutes, codes, or regulations regarding the emergency care of these persons. In New York State, a person "found to be incapacitated . . . to the degree that he or she may endanger self, other persons, or property, . . . may be retained in such facility or services over his or her objection until no longer incapacitated to such degree or no longer than a period of 24 hours . . ." (*New York Official Compilation,* 1982). In the case of Mr. B., he readily agreed to stay overnight. The psychiatrist can more reliably evaluate the patient once the patient is sober, as was the case with Mr. B. During this reevaluation, the psychiatrist determined that the patient was severely depressed and suicidal and met the criteria for emergency psychiatric hospitalization.

## DECISION TO HOSPITALIZE PSYCHIATRICALLY

Clinicians providing emergency psychiatric services are faced with making two crucial clinical–legal decisions regarding each patient: Does the patient require hospitalization and, if the patient refuses admission, does he or she meet the criteria for civil commitment (Appelbaum & Gutheil, 1991)? As background for this subject, it is important for the emergency room clinician to understand that commitment rules and regulations are continually changing—though, as Miller (1991) has written, these changes now occur in a more "evolutionary manner, in contrast to the revolution of the 1970's" (p. 161). Moreover, these commitment statutes vary somewhat from state to state. Significantly, with the current emphasis on community-based treatment, the general hospital emergency room is where most initial evaluations for involuntary commitments take place (Segal, Watson, Goldfinger, & Averbuck, 1988). But it should also be noted that, in recent years, there has been a trend toward voluntary admissions, which account for some 70% of all current hospitalizations in the country (Winick, 1991).

Although a detailed history of the alternating swing of the pendulum between *parens patriae* (the state acting as a beneficent parent) and the state's "police powers" as the basis of commitment laws is beyond the scope of this chapter, certain points that seem of particular relevance to the emergency room clinician will be discussed. With the passage of the Lanterman-Petris-Short Act in 1969, California became the first state to restrict involuntary hospitalization to dangerousness and to the "gravely disabled." The latter category is essentially a variation of the dangerous-to-self criterion. In 1972, the court ruled in *Lessard v. Schmidt* that the Wisconsin statute on civil commitment was unconstitutional because, without a finding of dangerousness to self or others, it was too vague to serve as the basis for depriving a person of his or her liberty through involuntary hospitalization. These events heralded the enactment, during the 1970s, by every state legislature except New York of commitment laws requiring a standard of dangerousness for involuntary psychiatric hospitalization. Recently New York State also added the dangerousness criterion for involuntary nonemergency admissions. The Certificate of Examining Physician in New York State requires that each of the two physicians in support of an application for nonemergency involuntary admission find that "this person has a mental illness for which care and treatment in a mental hospital is appropriate; as a result of this mental illness, this person poses a substantial threat of harm to him/herself or others (substantial threat of harm to him/herself shall include the inability to safely survive in the community); and hospitalization can reasonably be expected to improve this person's condition or at least prevent his/her deterioration."

It should be noted that the "care and treatment" point may be interpreted as retention of the *parens patriae* aspect of the procedure, the "inability to safely survive in the community" note as a gravely disabled component, and the "expected to improve condition" provision as justification for deprivation of liberty for treatment purposes in contrast to punitive purposes in criminal detention. Appelbaum and Gutheil (1991) have emphasized that "the difference between a dangerous psychotic person and a dangerous non-mentally ill criminal is that hospitalization of the former is likely to benefit him . . . . *Parens patriae* rationales are therefore inherent in any system of commitment, even one limited to dangerous persons" (p. 47).

The basic question of what is meant by "dangerousness" continues to generate much debate. Should it be interpreted in the narrow or broad sense? Is it essentially a public policy consideration? Fisher, Pierce, and Appelbaum (1988) have indicated that, though civil commitment standards tend to be interpreted strictly, the areas of ambiguity in the language of commitment statutes such as the grave-disability component have allowed mental health professionals some discretion to "enlarge the category of conditions that can justify commitment" (p. 712).

Because the result of the psychiatric examination may be involuntary civil commitment with the attendant deprivation of liberty, a seemingly important question is whether or not the patient has the right to remain silent as protected by the Fifth Amendment against self-incrimination. Griffith and Griffith (1982) discuss this issue and conclude that, while the Fifth Amendment privilege against self-incrimination is not necessarily limited to evidence produced in criminal proceedings, "there has been no real movement to apply it to the area of civil commitment . . . due in large measure to the theory of benevolence and paternalism which pervades the commitment process" (p. 296).

As many clinicians involved in the process will confirm, managing the involuntary civil commitment may be a very difficult professional undertaking (Knapp & VandeCreek, 1987). Under some of the most difficult and stressful clinical circumstances, the mental health professional is required to make what amount to psychiatric–legal decisions that conceivably could have dire consequences. Of great concern to many mental health professionals is possible tort liability for their decisions. Knapp and VandeCreek (1987) have reviewed some of the major areas of tort liability in such situations; these areas include malpractice, malicious persecution, false imprisonment, and abuse of process. They conclude that although "there have been several cases in which mental health professionals have been held liable for negligent behavior . . . the law recognizes the difficulties in civil commitment decisions and protects conscientious professionals who follow the letter and spirit of the law" (p. 651).

With regard to voluntary psychiatric hospitalizations, the 1990 U.S. Supreme Court decision in *Zinermon v. Burch* has generated considerable discussion. In that decision, the Supreme Court ruled that a mentally ill person who was incompetent to give informed consent but was admitted to a state hospital under voluntary admission procedures could bring a federal civil rights suit against those state officials involved in the admission. Appelbaum (1990) observes that the decision seems to imply that patients seeking voluntary admission should be screened for their competence to give informed consent prior to hospitalization. Winick (1991) points out that the Court's language could have negative therapeutic consequences because a significant number of patients admitted voluntarily would probably not be considered competent in a traditional sense. Thus many of these patients could be deprived of the advantages of voluntary admission, including earlier treatment intervention and less stigmatization. Winick emphasizes, however, that much of the Court's language in *Zinermon* is "dicta," meaning that it consists of unduly broad statements that go beyond the facts in the case. Consequently, Winick advises state legislatures to be cautious about making broad changes in their statutes on voluntary admission based on language whose implications have not been fully considered by the Court.

## Case 3: Involuntary Civil Commitment

Ms. C., a 34-year-old single, unemployed woman residing with her mother and subsisting on welfare, was brought by her mother into the emergency room of a general hospital in New York State in the late afternoon. The mother requested that her daughter be admitted to the psychiatric unit because of a recent worsening of her chronic mental illness. According to the mother, for the past several weeks the daughter had started to talk increasingly to herself, not to wash or take care of herself, to complain of hearing voices and that people were talking about her, and to leave the apartment at all hours of the day or night, twice having had to be brought back by relatives. Ms. C. has been known to be mentally ill since her first psychiatrical hospitalization at the age of 22. Subsequent to that event, she has had numerous other hospitalizations, generally when she stops taking her medication and attending the aftercare clinic. This time the patient had not taken any of her prescribed Haldol medication for two months, and still refuses medication, as well as to attend the clinic, because she considers it no longer necessary. The mother is worried that her daughter's condition will continue to deteriorate, as has happened many times in the past; she says that the only thing that helped her daughter in the past was to hospitalize her and force her to take medication.

The clinician interviewed the patient and found her to be alert and fully oriented, but quite suspicious and only minimally cooperative. She acknowledged experiencing auditory hallucinations of a woman's voice talking and calling her bad names, and that she had a paranoid fear of being harmed. Her affect was flattened and sometimes inappropriate. Speech was at times irrelevant, with mild derailment. She flatly denied having any suicidal or homicidal ideation. Insight and judgment were defective. She insisted that there was nothing seriously wrong with her, and that she was tired of her nagging mother who would not allow her to be more independent and to go out by herself. She refused to consider taking any medication, returning to her aftercare clinic, or entering the psychiatric unit as a voluntary admission.

The psychiatrist explained to the mother in private that her daughter did not meet the criteria for an emergency admission, but could be admitted on a two-physician certificate with the mother as petitioner. The mother readily agreed to be the petitioner; the psychiatrist and another physician who examined the patient filled out the Certificate of Examining Physician, and the patient was admitted to the psychiatric unit on an involuntary basis.

## Discussion of Case 3

The psychiatric–legal questions of whether the patient required hospitalization and whether the patient met the criteria for involuntary hospitalization in New York State were both affirmed. The psychiatrist determined that the patient had a mental illness that posed a substantial threat to herself as a result of her erratic behavior, particularly her inability to care for herself and her going out at all hours in an unsafe neighborhood. Considering her history, hospitalization conceivably could improve her condition, and because she refused to take medication or to attend her mental health clinic, there was no alternative form of treatment. It should be noted that the New York State commitment statutes require two examining physicians to complete the commitment certificate. An examining physician is one who is duly licensed to practice medicine. And it should be emphasized that New York State involuntary commitment procedures do not require, as do many other jurisdictions, that the patient be taken to a designated community agency for independent evaluation or subjected to an adversarial procedure at a judicial hearing or some other such evaluation. In New York State, the patient on admission is given a patient's bill of rights and access to legal counsel in the form of a Mental Hygiene Legal Service attorney to assist, if needed, in contesting the involuntary hospitalization. Because the commitment criteria vary from state to state, it is incumbent on the clinician to become familiar with his or her state regulations.

## EMERGENCY ROOM ASSESSMENT AND MANAGEMENT OF VIOLENCE

The assessment and management of violent patients constitute one of the greatest challenges facing clinicians in the emergency room. Since "violence" is a generic term that characterizes a range of behaviors, but is neither a diagnostic entity, a mental disorder, nor a "characterological style," not all violent patients can be treated in the same way (Reid, 1989). Generally, in order to initiate appropriate treatment, the clinician needs to conduct an adequate clinical evaluation of the underlying pathology. Dubin (1981) lists some diagnostic groups that predispose the patient to violence as follows: drug or alcohol intoxication, drug or alcohol withdrawal, acute organic brain syndrome (delirium), acute psychosis, paranoid character, borderline personality, antisocial personality, and other diagnostic categories, such as temporal lobe epilepsy, passive-aggressive personality, and pathological intoxication.

Dubin also cites Hackett's guide to behavioral clues that are indicative of a patient's potential for violence, including the patient's posture, speech, and motor activity. Yet, clinicians must be able to make a rapid assessment and take decisive action in the management of an acute violent episode. This action necessarily must take precedence over the diagnosis and specific treatment of underlying pathology. Depending on the situation, management may include verbal, pharmacological, and restraining intervention.

Because of the possibility of delirium or of a toxic metabolic state, physical restraints employed as a "holding action" to enable an emergency medical examination should precede medication (Soloff, 1987). In fact, Soloff emphasizes that the clinician can avoid the risks of rapid tranquilization entirely if, at his or her discretion, the clinician uses physical restraints appropriately in emergency situations. In all cases, the clinician should carefully document the justification for his or her course of action.

Clinically relevant guidelines for the psychiatric uses of seclusion and restraint were formulated by a task force of the American Psychiatric Association (APA) (Tardiff, 1984). Basically, the nurse or some other professional staff member usually initiates the hospital emergency restraining procedure that is in conformity with state regulations, and notifies the physician. The physician is required personally to see the patient as soon as possible. Appelbaum (1987) points out that the clinician is obligated to respect two sets of patients' rights, the "right to be free of violent assault" and the "right to be free of unnecessary restraint"—rights that "are at times in conflict with each other" (p. 549).

As an important educational measure, emergency room clinicians should familiarize themselves with the current research pertaining to the prediction of violent behavior. Although the so-called first generation of research studies had indicated that clinicians had no particular expertise in predicting future violent behavior, a second generation of research and theory on predicting violence has begun to emerge (Monahan, 1984). Whereas the first generation of research was involved with clinical predictions of patients' potential for violence in long-term custodial institutions, the new research has focused on other settings of predictions (such as in short-term community settings), and also has emphasized actuarial methods of prediction. Thus Monahan (1984) expresses a guarded optimism that the ceiling level of accuracy of clinical prediction "may be closer to 50% than to 5% among some groups of clinical interest" (p. 11). The American Civil Liberties Union had asserted that psychiatrists and psychologists were inaccurate in their predictions of violent behavior about 95% of the time. Monahan claims that the new scholarship on violence is much more inclined to review the "public policies that rely on prediction in terms of relative rather than absolute moral and political values" (p. 11).

In recent years, considerable research has been focusing on finding clinically relevant variables to predict violent behavior in order to justify the criteria of dangerousness for civil commitment. In this regard, Beck, White, and Gage (1991) recently published the results of their study on whether there are certain clinical and demographic features that distinguish dangerous from nondangerous patients evaluated in a psychiatric emergency service of a city hospital, and whether there are certain variables that correlate with hospitalization. They found that the patients who were hospitalized were more likely to have engaged in recent violent acts, and to have been brought into the emergency room in restraints by the police, or were psychotic. Beck et al. (1991) concluded that "state variables are associated with patient dangerousness and disposition on a psychiatric setting; demographics are not" (p. 1564).

With regard to the Tarasoff responsibility or duty of mental health professionals to "protect" potential victims from harm committed by their patients, emergency room psychiatrists are just as vulnerable to suits as psychiatrists would be in other settings "if they wrongfully violate confidentiality or inadequately attend to protecting potential victims of their patients" (White & Beck, 1990, p. 43). Consequently, Appelbaum (1988) has expressed concern that this fear of liability has influenced some psychiatrists to hospitalize patients who may not be mentally ill, solely to prevent them from committing violence. This amounts to the "creation of a de facto system of preventive detention" (p. 779).

In addition to all these considerations, clinicians should be aware that the countertransference reactions these patients evoke in the clinician are a major interference in the evaluation and management of violent patients. Lion and Pasternack (1973) use Colby's definition of countertransference: "any emotional reaction that the clinician has toward the patient" (p. 297). These reactions can range from anger and helplessness, which increase the clinician's fear that the patient will do something terrible, to denial as a defense against anxiety, which results in the clinician's not eliciting sufficient data on the patient's violence potential, and at times even results in the clinician's identifying with aggressive patients in ward settings. Rada (1981) has pointed out that, just as in the past some clinicians were hesitant to inquire directly about the patient's suicide potential, some clinicians today tend to experience denial and thus avoid direct questioning about the patient's potential for violence.

## Case 4: The Violent Patient

Mr. D., a 29-year-old homeless man, was brought handcuffed by police officers into the emergency room of a general hospital; he was in a highly agitated state and his breath smelled of alcohol. He was reported to have engaged a shopper in a supermarket in a heated argument, and then to shout obscenities at other people and to complain that everybody was trying to cheat him. When the police officers arrived, he begged them to shoot him. They restrained him and brought him to the hospital.

When an attempt was made to examine him physically, he refused to allow it and became combative. The psychiatrist interviewed him and found him to be agitated, with the smell of alcohol on his breath, only partially oriented, suspicious, and with paranoid delusions of people wanting to harm him because they were jealous of him. He said he was tired of it all and wanted to die. When asked specifically about having homicidal thoughts, he acknowledged that he had been thinking of killing a former girlfriend, whom he accused of cheating on him and leaving him for another man three years earlier. Upon further questioning, he became increasingly irritable, hostile, and agitated, and refused to continue the interview. His agitation escalated rapidly to the point that he began to threaten the staff with violence.

The psychiatrist ordered that the patient be restrained. This was accomplished with considerable difficulty because the patient continued to resist violently. The psychiatrist also ordered a small dose of Haldol. Mr. D. was placed on constant observation with a trained psychiatric technician. The patient calmed down considerably within 30 minutes. As a result of these measures, the medical internist was able to examine him physically and to draw blood for laboratory studies. Mr. D. went into a deep sleep and awoke six hours later. He was reinterviewed, at which time he gave additional information about multiple past psychiatric hospitalizations and episodic alcohol abuse. Although he was now fully oriented and no longer agitated, he continued to have paranoid delusions and suicidal and homicidal ideations; consequently, he was admitted to the psychiatric unit on an emergency status. The psychiatrist documented his entire clinical encounter with the patient on the patient's chart; he also contacted the ward psychiatrist and informed him about the patient's homicidal ideation.

## Discussion of Case 4

Among the most difficult psychiatric–legal decisions that the clinician is required to make in the emergency room are those pertaining to the acutely violent patient. As a case in point, the patient described above was intoxicated, was severely agitated and combative, and represented an immediate danger to self and staff. Despite the clinician's inability to examine the patient physically, there was an urgent need to control his violent behavior. Rapidly assessing the situation, the clinician ordered physical restraints. The use of mechanical restraints is often the first line of treatment for an out-of-control psychiatric patient (Telintelo, Kuhlman, & Winget, 1983). Physical restraints ordered by a psychiatrist, however, generally require a more stringent set of guidelines (as indicated in the APA task force guidelines) than when ordered by the medical internist for a medical emergency such as acute delirium. It is important that staff members who provide constant observation of patients not be untrained security guards, but technically trained personnel. Because the patient had the smell of alcohol on his breath and presumably was intoxicated, judicious use of medication was an absolute necessity. In this case, each of these treatments (physical restraints, observation by a psychiatric technician, and a small dose of medication) was performed on an emergency basis and was duly documented.

The psychiatric–legal decision to hospitalize the patient as an emergency was based on the patient's paranoid delusions, which were accompanied by suicidal and homicidal ideations. The psychiatrist determined that the patient represented an immediate danger to self and others and thus met the criteria of dangerousness for emergency admission to the psychiatric unit. Since the patient had not acted on his homicidal ideation for three years, and because the patient claimed that he did not know the whereabouts of his ex-girlfriend, the psychiatrist decided to document the patient's homicidal ideation clearly on the chart, and to inform the treating psychiatrist on the inpatient service about the matter. This was done to ensure that the treating psychiatrist would be aware of the patient's homicidal ideation and so would continue to reevaluate the patient.

## EMERGENCY ROOM EVALUATION OF THE SUICIDAL PATIENT

The evaluation of suicidal patients in the emergency room is another of the clinician's most difficult duties. Because suicide is such a significant health problem—it ranks eighth among all causes of death in this country (Goldstein, Black, Nasrallah, & Winokur, 1991)—clinicians should inquire about suicidal potential in every psychiatric patient they encounter in the emergency room. There is no definitive way to assess suicidal potential in the individual case aside from the clinician's specifically eliciting the patient's self-report or intent or plan, information that some seriously suicidal patients may be determined to withhold. Therefore, in a situation in which the clinician suspects that vital information about suicidal intention is being withheld, it is absolutely necessary that he or she make every effort to obtain any substantiating information possible, with or without the patient's permission. In this situation, the clinician should not be concerned about breaching confidentiality.

Research on the subject of suicide has been attempting to identify for the clinician generally useful risk factors. Many researchers have pointed out that more than 90% of suicide victims were psychiatrically ill immediately prior to their suicidal act (Goldstein et al., 1991). Goldstein and colleagues consider depression, alcoholism, and schizophrenia to be the most important factors contributing to suicide, and list additional risk factors as "male gender . . . increasing age, living alone, any marital status other than married and living with spouse, a history of early parental loss, presence of suicidal ideation during index episode of psychiatric illness, history of prior suicide attempts, racial/ethnic identity other than black, abnormal personality, physical illness, . . . hopelessness, and, especially for alcoholics, recent interpersonal loss" (p. 418). However, these authors caution that the use of these risk factors in predicting suicide will produce a considerable number of false-positive results. In their study of a group of patients at high risk for suicide among patients admitted to a tertiary-care hospital for affective disorders, Goldstein et al. (1991) concluded that, though the index of suspicion should be high with patients having several known risk factors for suicide, the health-care professional's knowledge about the individual patient remains "the best tool for the prevention of suicides" (pp. 421–422).

Murphy (1986) emphasizes that, because of the relationship between suicide and such psychiatric illnesses as depression, alcoholism, organic brain syndrome, and schizophrenia, the clinician should examine carefully for a psychiatric diagnosis of significance as a risk factor for suicide, and should be especially concerned about depression and alcoholism. Murphy also points out that there is a difference between seriously suicidal patients, who are predominantly male and are commonly suffering from a psychiatric illness such as affective disorder or alcoholism, and suicide attempters, who are predominantly women who act impulsively with a purpose to survive, but under changed circumstances, and whose act mostly represents a cry for help. Nevertheless, Murphy acknowledges that "in the final analysis, suicide attempters do, as a group, carry increased risk for suicide" (p. 314).

Appelbaum and Gutheil (1991) point out that in the assessment of the suicidal patient, the clinician must clarify the factors that contribute to the urgency of the present situation, including "risk factors and resource factors, external and internal" (p. 60). These authors stress that, once the clinician makes a determination that a serious suicidal risk exists, he or she must act decisively and "take over" responsibility to prevent delay and ensure that the patient is observed and protected from attempting suicide in the emergency room itself.

## Case 5: The Suicidal Patient

Ms. E., a 20-year-old single woman employed as a cashier in a supermarket and residing with her parents, was brought by ambulance to the emergency room of a general hospital after she had swallowed about seven of her mother's pain pills earlier that evening. She was accompanied by her mother, who reported that her daughter had gone into the bathroom, where she swallowed the pills, and then came out complaining of feeling nauseated and admitted to what she had done. Ms. E.'s mother said she believed that her daughter had been feeling depressed about a recent breakup with her boyfriend.

The medical staff in the emergency room telephoned the poison control bureau and started immediate, vigorous treatment. Ms. E. was kept overnight in the emergency room and was determined the following morning to be stable medically. A psychiatric consultation was requested to reevaluate whether she was suicidal and in need of psychiatric hospitalization.

The psychiatrist interviewed the patient and found her to be alert, cooperative, fully oriented, and without any evidence of psychosis. She was slightly depressed, but she expressed regret over what she had done and insisted that she had not really wanted to kill herself, but only to get away from her problem. She said that she had never done anything like this before, nor would she ever do it again. She related that she had been trying to get over the breakup with her boyfriend for the past week, but when her mother had mentioned him and asked how she was feeling, she had felt overwhelmed and in need of escaping. She now recognized that the breakup was probably for the better as they were not really suitable for each other, and said that she wanted to get on with her life. She readily agreed to have the psychiatrist speak to her mother about the situation, and also to accept referral for further outpatient counseling. After speaking with the patient's mother, who expressed eagerness to be of support to her daughter, the psychiatrist decided to release Ms. E., and gave her a return appointment to the mental health clinic for the next day.

### Discussion of Case 5

In this case, the psychiatric–legal decision not to hospitalize the patient psychiatrically followed a careful assessment of the patient's suicidal potential. In this assessment, the psychiatrist considered the seriousness of the suicide attempt. Supporting his decision to release the patient were her willingness to accept further counseling, the presence of a support system in the form of an understanding family, the patient's diagnosis (not psychotic or severely depressed), the lack of an alcohol/substance-abuse history, and the absence of previous suicide attempts. Importantly, the patient did not fulfill the criteria for emergency or nonemergency commitment to a psychiatric hospital. She did not want to sign herself into a hospital voluntarily; she wanted treatment as an outpatient.

## CONCLUSION

Clinicians providing care in emergency rooms should be mindful that while they necessarily must be aggressive in attending to the emergent needs of the patient, they also are obligated to take into consideration the patient's basic rights. Thus the prudent emergency room clinician should decide to hospitalize patients involuntarily only after considering whether it is clearly warranted, to medicate or restrain patients judiciously and only with proper justification, and to breach confidentiality only when indicated and only to the extent that is absolutely necessary. In this way, the patient can get the right treatment without losing his or her rights as an individual.

## REFERENCES

American Psychiatric Association. (1987). *Diagnostic and statistical manual of mental disorders* (3d ed., rev.). Washington, DC: American Psychiatric Press.

Ananth, J., Vandewater, S., Kanmal, M., Brodsky, A., Gamal, R., & Miller, M. (1989). Mixed diagnosis of substance abuse in psychiatric patients. *Hospital and Community Psychiatry, 40,* 297–299.

Appelbaum, P. S. (1987). Legal aspects of violence by psychiatric patients. In K. Tardiff (Section Ed.), *Annual review: Vol. 6. Violence and the violent patient* (pp. 549–564). Washington, DC: American Psychiatric Press.

Appelbaum, P. S. (1988). The new preventive detention: psychiatry's problematic responsibility for the control of violence. *American Journal of Psychiatry, 145,* 779–785.

Appelbaum, P. S. (1990). Voluntary hospitalization and due process: The dilemma of *Zinermon v. Burch. Hospital and Community Psychiatry, 41,* 1059–1060.

Appelbaum, P. S., & Gutheil, T. G. (1991). *Clinical handbook of psychiatry and the law* (2d ed.). Baltimore, MD: Williams & Wilkins.

Bassuk, E. L., & Gerson, S. (1979). Into the breach: Emergency psychiatry in the general hospital. *General Hospital Psychiatry, 1,* 31–45.

Beck, J. C., White, K. A., & Gage, B. (1991). Emergency psychiatric assessment of violence. *American Journal of Psychiatry, 148,* 1562–1565.

Dubin, W. R. (1981). Evaluating and managing the violent patient. *Annals of Emergency Medicine, 10,* 481–484.

Dubin, W. R., & Weiss, K. J. (1986). Emergency psychiatry. In J. L. Houpt & H. K. H. Brodie (Eds.), *Psychiatry: Vol. 3. Consultation–liaison psychiatry and behavioral medicine* (pp. 147–161). New York: Basic Books.

Fisher, W. H., Pierce, G. I., & Appelbaum, P. S. (1988). How flexible are our civil commitment statutes? *Hospital and Community Psychiatry, 39,* 711–712.

Fogel, B. S., Mills, M. J., & Landen, J. E. (1986). Legal aspects of the treatment of delirium. *Hospital and Community Psychiatry, 37,* 154–158.

Goldstein, R. B., Black, D. W., Nasrallah, A., & Winokur, G. (1991). The prediction of suicide: Sensitivity, specificity, and predictive value of a multivariate model applied to suicide among 1906 patients with affective disorder. *Archives of General Psychiatry, 48,* 418–422.

Griffith, E. J., & Griffith, E. H. (1982). The patient's right to protection against self-incrimination during the psychiatric examination. *Toledo Law Review, 13,* 269–298.

Hall, R. C. W., & Beresford, T. P. (1986). Psychiatric manifestations of physical illness. In J. L. Houpt & H. K. H. Brodie (Eds.), *Psychiatry: Vol. 3. Consultation–liaison psychiatry and behavioral medicine* (pp. 95–112). New York: Basic Books.

Hall, R. C. W., Popkin, M. K., Devaul, R. A., Faillace, L. A., & Stickney, S. K. (1978). Physical illness presenting as psychiatric disease. *Archives of General Psychiatry, 35,* 1315–1320.

Halleck, S. L. (1980). *Law in the practice of psychiatry: A handbook for clinicians.* New York: Plenum.

Johnson, D. A. W. (1968). The evaluation of routine physical examination in psychiatric cases. *Practitioner, 200,* 686–691.

Julavits, W. F. (1983). Legal issues in emergency psychiatry. In S. M. Soreff (Ed.), *The psychiatric clinics of North America: Vol. 6. Emergency psychiatry* (pp. 335–345). Philadelphia, PA: Saunders.

Knapp, S., & VandeCreek, L. (1987). A review of tort liability in involuntary civil commitment. *Hospital and Community Psychiatry, 38,* 648–665.

Leeman, C. P. (1975). Diagnostic errors in emergency room medicine: Physical illness in patients labeled "psychiatric" and vice versa. *International Journal of Psychiatry in Medicine, 6,* 533–540.

Lehman, A. F., Meyers, C. P., & Corty, E. (1989). Assessment and classification of patients with psychiatric and substance abuse syndromes. *Hospital and Community Psychiatry, 40,* 1019–1025.

*Lessard v. Schmidt,* 340 F.Supp 1078, E.D. Wis. (1972).

Linn, L. (1971). Emergency room psychiatry: A gateway to community medicine. *Mount Sinai Journal of Medicine, 38,* 110–120.

Lion, J. R., & Pasternack, S. A. (1973). Countertransference reactions to violent patients. *American Journal of Psychiatry, 130,* 207–210.

Melinek, M., Bluestone, H., & Steinmuller, R. (1983). The psychiatrist as a "presence": Possible effects on emergency room staff attitudes. *General Hospital Psychiatry, 6,* 77–79.

Miller, R. D. (1991). Involuntary civil commitment. In R. I. Simon (Ed.), *Review of clinical psychiatry and the law* (Vol. 2, pp. 95–172). Washington, DC: American Psychiatric Press.

Monahan, J. (1984). The prediction of violent behavior: Toward a second generation of theory and policy. *American Journal of Psychiatry, 141,* 10–15.

Murphy, G. E. (1986). Suicide and attempted suicide. In J. E. Helzer & S. B. Guze (Eds.), *Psychiatry: Vol. 2. Psychoses, affective disorders and dementia* (pp. 299–315). New York: Basic Books.

New York Official Compilation of Codes, Rules, and Regulations, tit. 14, sec. 304.4 (1982).

Rada, R. T. (1981). The violent patient: Rapid assessment and management. *Psychosomatics, 22,* 101–105.

Reid, W. H. (1989). Treatment of violent patients: Concerns for the psychiatrist. In W. H. Sledge (Section Ed.), *Annual review: Vol. 8. Difficult situations in clinical practice* (pp. 549–562). Washington, DC: American Psychiatric Press.

Segal, S. P., Watson, M. A., Goldfinger, S. M., & Averbuck, D. S. (1988). Civil commitment in the psychiatric emergency room, Part I. The assessment of dangerousness by emergency room clinicians. *Archives of General Psychiatry, 45,* 748–752.

Soloff, P. H. (1987). Emergency management of violent patients. In K. Tardiff (Section Ed.), *Annual review: Vol. 6. Violence and the violent patient* (pp. 510–536). Washington, DC: American Psychiatric Press.

Swartz, M. S. (1987). What constitutes a psychiatric emergency: Clinical and legal dimensions. *Bulletin of the American Academy of Psychiatry and the Law, 15,* 57–68.

Szuster, R. R., Schanbacher, B. L., & McCann, S. C. (1990). Characteristics of psychiatric emergency room patients with alcohol- or drug-induced disorders. *Hospital and Community Psychiatry, 41,* 1342–1345.

Tancredi, L. S. (1982). Emergency psychiatry and crisis intervention: Some legal and ethical issues. *Psychiatric Annals, 12,* 779–806.

Tardiff, K. (Ed.). (1984). *The psychiatric uses of seclusion and restraint.* Washington, DC: American Psychiatric Press.

Telintelo, S., Kuhlman, T. L., & Winget, C. (1983). A study of the use of restraint in a psychiatric emergency room. *Hospital and Community Psychiatry, 34,* 164–165.

Weissberg, M. P. (1979). Emergency room medical clearance: An educational problem. *American Journal of Psychiatry, 136,* 787–790.

White, K. A., & Beck, J. C. (1990). The duty to protect in emergency psychiatry. In J. C. Beck (Ed.), *Confidentiality versus the duty to protect: Foreseeable harm in the practice of psychiatry* (pp. 43–53). Washington, DC: American Psychiatric Press.

Winick, B. J. (1991). Voluntary hospitalization after *Zinermon v. Burch. Psychiatric Annals, 21,* 584–589.

*Zinermon v. Burch,* 110 S.Ct. 975 (1990).

# 4

# Retention and Treatment Issues on the Psychiatric Inpatient Unit

## STEPHEN RACHLIN

General hospital psychiatric services care for a wide variety of patients, at least some of whom will be retained on an involuntary basis. It is, therefore, imperative that the psychiatrist understand the legal implications of such status. There are clear-cut variations among states in how the law is written and how it operates. Nothing can really replace knowledge of the ins and outs of civil commitment statutes, regulations, and practices. Similarly, some patients may need to be treated despite their objections, and just how this is to be handled also requires specific understanding of what needs to be done in a particular jurisdiction.

Obviously, no single chapter can do justice to the differences throughout the United States in how psychiatric units operate within boundaries that give due respect to patients' rights. For each of the major divisions, civil commitment and the right to refuse treatment, the following sets forth relevant and generalizable developments in the law, followed by a summary of research on the topic, and then by a set of informal guidelines for the practical application of medicolegal principles.

Of necessity, this chapter is an overview, and is not intended to be exhaustive. The choice of the literature is somewhat selective, with an attempt to focus on material that should be relatively accessible to the general hospital psychiatrist. Readers who want additional clinically oriented information should consult Miller's book (1987) or the appropriate sections of either Simon's text (1992) or that by Appelbaum and Gutheil (1991). A fine legal reference is the three-volume work by Perlin (1989), which is updated with annual supplements.

## CIVIL COMMITMENT

### Developments in the Law

Involuntary psychiatric hospitalization includes both emergency admission and longer-term retention. The latter generally requires a judicial proceeding, and is what is usually meant by the term "civil commitment." It is to be distinguished from commitment under one or another provision of criminal law, a subject that will not be discussed here.

Given that hospitalization restricts physical freedoms, it is legally considered a deprivation of liberty, an act for which the Constitution demands due process of law. This concept involves striking a balance between what is to be lost and the fairness with which government goes about taking it away. Hardly a fixed notion, determining how much process is due in any particular situation is the proper business of lawmakers, ultimately to be determined and interpreted by courts.

The term "procedural due process" refers to the rules under which the deprivation is made. It includes, but is not limited to, such things as notice, a hearing, right to counsel, and trial by jury. Substantive due process, on the other hand, pertains to the standards and criteria according to which the decision is to be made.

There are two substantive principles by which involuntary hospitalization of the mentally ill is legally sanctioned. The first is called *parens patriae,* literally, the State as father, and calls into play the obligation of government to care for those who cannot do so for themselves. It is, in the psychiatric context, designed to benefit the committed person. Second, there is the police power of the state, which enables government to act to protect society from danger. Clinically, it translates as removing the so-called dangerous mentally ill from our collective midst. There is no bright line separating *parens patriae* from police power in day-to-day practice, but the distinction can be drawn on paper.

Hospitalization under police power would require overt evidence of danger to others as a result of mental illness. An essential ingredient, therefore, would be the accurate prediction or reasonable presumption of dangerousness. Suicidality is obviously dangerous to oneself, and so it is, at least in part, a police power standard. However, it also encompasses an element of *parens patriae,* as does the concept of grave disability, by which is meant that the individual, because of mental illness, is unable to provide for such basic needs as food, clothing, or shelter. The most conservative *parens patriae* criterion, based on a somewhat dated model, is a simple need for hospital-level care and treatment as a result of mental illness.

During the decade of the 1970s, most states legislatively changed their civil commitment statutes in the direction of requiring a finding of dangerousness, in other words, the police power standard. This was particularly true vis-à-vis extended, as opposed to emergency, hospitalization. Many similar changes came about through the process of litigation pursued by civil libertarians. Those who went to court to challenge hospitalization laws were successful more often than not. This group of lawyers, labeled paternalistic libertarians by Miller (1985), believed that they knew best what patients wanted and what was in their interest.

This brief discussion hardly does justice to a very complicated series of issues (Rachlin, 1983). The end result was a significant philosophical (as well as legal) shift from the acceptance of psychiatric hospitalization under *parens patriae* to the requirement that it be under police powers, with major procedural protections for the proposed patient. Society has chosen to place great emphasis on individual freedoms (Hoge, Appelbaum, & Geller, 1989). The irony in overturning need-for-treatment standards at the same time in history that effective treatments became available is pointed out by Miller (1987).

Today, in virtually all jurisdictions, civil commitment requires the presence of a mental illness, coupled with one or more of dangerousness to others, dangerousness to self, or grave disability. It must be mentioned that the purported danger should be a result of the mental illness, not simply a phenomenon that coexists with it. Even these common words are not easy to define: Perlin (1989) uses the term "elusive" in referring to a definition of mental illness and "vexing" to describe attempts to clarify dangerousness.

The prediction of dangerousness is not something for which clinicians claim great skill. However, the most operative fact in the context of involuntary psychiatric hospitalization is that danger does not necessarily mean actual violence. We all know this, and need to keep it in mind when considering the commitment of a patient. It was given recognition by the U.S. Supreme Court in a case involving an insanity acquittee (*Jones v. United States*, 1983).

That same court held that a state "cannot confine without more a nondangerous individual who is capable of surviving safely in freedom by himself or with the help of willing and responsible family members or friends" (*O'Connor v. Donaldson*, 1975). In so saying, however, the justices went on to add, "A person is literally dangerous to himself if for physical or other reasons he is helpless to avoid the hazards of freedom." Indeed, courts have not been overly rigid in their interpretation of what is necessary and sufficient for a finding of dangerousness. In another article (Rachlin, 1987), I collected a series of a dozen appellate court decisions spanning seven states wherein, for example, threats were accepted as evidence and comments to the effect that one need not wait for bloodshed, even in the case of an overt-act requirement, were made.

### Research Results

A steady stream of empirical literature attests that psychiatrists (and other clinicians) are able to practice effectively within the dangerousness standard, especially as it includes grave disability implying a danger to oneself. Schwartz, Appelbaum, and Kaplan (1984) studied decision making in the context of whether or not to commit voluntary patients requesting their release and found a strong correlation between legally relevant factors and criteria and medical action: doctors conformed to the dangerousness requirements of the commitment law. In another series, threats without action were common indicators of dangerousness, and this standard did not have a deleterious effect on the commitment process (Hiday & Smith, 1987).

Segal and colleagues (Segal, Watson, Goldfinger, & Averbuck, 1988) demonstrated a positive relationship between severe major

mental illness and a perception of fitting the dangerousness requirement of the law. Another study found that the judicial variables
(those the judge would have to use in making a determination) had
the highest order of correlation with the actual clinical conclusion
(Bursztajn, Gutheil, Hamm, Brodsky, & Mills, 1988). In looking at
the decision to hospitalize from the emergency room, a Pittsburgh
group (Cleveland, Mulvey, Appelbaum, & Lidz, 1989; Lidz, Mulvey,
Appelbaum, & Cleveland, 1989) found very few patients who were
highly in need of hospitalization, but who did not meet statutory
standards, and the clinicians had reasonably well-shared notions
about dangerousness. McFarland and co-workers (McFarland,
Faulkner, Bloom, Hallaux, & Bray, 1989) showed a similar influence
of concepts of inability to care for basic needs and dangerousness
among mental health professionals (and judges). Using vignettes,
Bagby and colleagues (Bagby, Thompson, Dickens, & Nohara, 1991)
established that the most important variables influencing their subjects (clinicians) were the legal standards and, to a lesser extent, the
presence of psychotic symptoms.

Several of the reports noted above also mentioned the relevance of
such clinical factors as severity of psychosis and the behavior produced
by the illness. Patients who are seriously and acutely disturbed are
hospitalized. Some vestiges of a *parens patriae* approach remain, but
there is no evidence of serious violations of patients' legal rights and
much data speaking to the fact that dangerousness criteria are used in
practice by psychiatrists and others involved in civil commitment.

Those of us who have in the past grown excessively fond of *parens
patriae* standards, as opposed to police power, need to be cognizant of
a series of studies that cast some doubt on the wisdom of this approach. In an often-cited article, Durham and LaFond (1985) looked
at the effect of Washington State's broadening the definition of grave
disability and adding property damage to what is encompassed by
harm. There was a drastic increase in the number of patients committed to state facilities, even in anticipation of the law's effective date.
Voluntary patients were essentially excluded from such hospital treatment, in what the researchers denominate as "the worst of both
worlds." The overcrowding ultimately led to court battles about
restricting admissions, with the state's highest court ruling that the

hospital had to take all referrals regardless of bed space or treatment resources.

Perhaps the best known *proposed* criteria for civil commitment with an overt *parens patriae* orientation are those that ultimately formed the basis for the American Psychiatric Association's model law (Stromberg & Stone, 1983). Hoge and colleagues (Hoge, Sachs, Appelbaum, Greer, & Gordon, 1988) found (perhaps surprisingly) that the dangerousness criteria were really less restrictive, because of the limitation imposed by that "Stone" standard which required an incompetent refusal of offered treatment prior to involuntary admission. Paternalism did not enlarge the scope of those at risk. Extending this work, Hoge, Appelbaum, and Greer (1989) affirmed that many people currently committable would not be under what turned out to be substantially narrower, albeit *parens patriae*–based, standards.

As the proverbial dust settles, several conclusions emerge. The most obvious is that both law and practice are in a state of evolution. Continuing study of the process is, because of its importance, a growth industry. Social scientists, with grant funding and multisite designs, will add to the database thus far generated primarily by clinicians (Miller, 1990). The direction of ongoing statutory modification appears to be toward broadening criteria and relaxing procedures somewhat (Hoge, Appelbaum, & Greer, 1989). It is likely that there will be an increasing number of patients admitted as gravely disabled (Perlin, 1989). And, as Appelbaum and Gutheil (1991) teach, *parens patriae* is inherent in any system of involuntary hospitalization because it is the availability of care and treatment that justifies the confinement of even the dangerous mentally ill.

**Putting Theory into Practice**

Armed with a theoretical understanding of the legal basis for civil commitment, and what the research shows, as outlined above, the psychiatrist or other clinician needs to know the substantive criteria enumerated by state statute in his or her jurisdiction, as well as the procedural rules and any local adaptations. But first and foremost, it cannot be overstated that the decision to proceed with civil commitment is a *clinical* one, to be made with the patient, his or her involved family, and the treatment team.

One's threshold for instituting the panoply of steps necessary to secure continued involuntary hospitalization must be psychiatrically realistic, and, while mindful of state standards, should not be set artificially high. Attempts to second-guess, in advance, what the outcome of a hearing might be are likely to be counterproductive. The first option, rather obviously, is to make all attempts, by whatever persuasive means are available therapeutically, to secure the patient's consent to remain in the hospital on a voluntary basis. A reasonable amount of time should be allowed for this process to take place.

Assuming that no agreement can be reached, then the legal route must be pursued. Hoge and co-workers (1989) caution that the manner in which commitment is handled is likely to have lasting effects on the patient's attitudes toward psychiatric treatment. Clearly, it represents an impasse in therapy; the patient should be told that it is the judge who will make the final decision in the matter (Simon, 1992). Interestingly, the ultimate authority of the judiciary is so ingrained in our society that only the patient unusually out of touch with reality will fail to grasp that point.

The atmosphere of a court, whether held at the hospital or at the courthouse, is strangely formal to the average clinician. For most of us, civil commitment hearings may be our only involvement with judges, judicial hearing officers, or even juries (depending on local statute and practice). Psychiatry and the law operate from very different conceptual models, only one of which will be detailed here (Gutheil, Rachlin, & Mills, 1985). The adversary system under which the court functions reflects the fact that there is a conflict that has not been able to be resolved by compromise or other negotiation. The attorneys, both for the hospital and for the patient, have an ethical obligation to present their facts in a way that makes their position look best. It cannot be thought for a moment that the patient's lawyer does not understand the hospital's point of view—he or she is there simply to contest retention by all legal means. Indeed, as Miller (1987) has shown, the way in which the lawyers for both sides do their jobs is a very important determinant of the ultimate outcome.

At the hearing, the patient is entitled to a host of procedural rights (Miller, 1987; Perlin, 1989). Among these are the right to be present and to cross-examine (through the lawyer) witnesses, including the psychiatrist or other testifying clinician. Thus the patient will hear the diagnosis and its basis. The astute clinician will have discussed this with the patient beforehand, both as part of therapy and to mitigate potential adverse consequences from learning unpleasant facts for the first time in a court. In some jurisdictions, the patient must be informed that what he or she tells the psychiatrist or clinical staff on the unit may be used in evidence against the patient at a commitment hearing, but this has been shown to have minimal influence over patients' willingness to talk (Miller, Maier, & Kaye, 1985).

Three standards of proof are recognized by the law. The first, preponderance of the evidence, represents anything over half. Second, clear and convincing is usually thought of as about 75% of the evidence. The final standard, beyond a reasonable doubt, used for criminal convictions, is considered to be about a 95% probability (in research terms, $p = .05$). The U.S. Supreme Court decided, in *Addington v. Texas* (1979), that the Constitution requires at least the level of clear and convincing for the liberty deprivation inherent in civil commitment. Some states, however, have opted for the higher standard of beyond a reasonable doubt. Lest this be considered a clinical impossibility, Appelbaum and Gutheil (1991) point out that it is only the existence of a risk that must be proved, not that an act of violence will take place. Our abilities to do this in the short term are probably adequate.

When testifying, the psychiatrist or other authorized clinician must present the facts leading to the diagnosis of mental illness and the circumstances yielding the conclusion that the patient meets the statutory standard of dangerousness, however defined. History, mental status, and observations constitute our data. Since commitment is designed, in part, to prevent violence, it would likely be acceptable (in appropriate circumstances) to show that since the symptoms of illness that led to the dangerous behavior that resulted in emergency detention are still present, the patient continues to pose a danger even though he or she has assaulted no one in the hospital. Or a demonstrated progression from agitation to abusiveness to threats to actions could buttress one's testimony. It is my belief that the psychiatrist should let it be known to the judge or other decision maker precisely how the patient is seen clinically and why the retention decision was made. Advance preparation with the hospital attorney will be very useful in this regard.

The quality of the presentation will go a long way toward assuring the desired outcome. We should have this clearly in mind, and avoid the temptation to let the court decide clinically ambiguous situations. Bursztajn and co-workers (Bursztajn, Gutheil, Mills, Hamm, & Brodsky, 1986) have shown that convincing psychiatric opinion has great strength in influencing judges' commitment decisions. They come to their conclusions much in the same way as we do to ours, and grant most petitions for continued hospitalization.

*Example*

A 48-year-old man, with a history of several prior hospitalizations and a diagnosis of bipolar disorder, was admitted after being brought in by the police because he threatened his landlady. Despite several weeks' treatment with adequate doses of lithium and an antipsychotic, he remained dysfunctional, expressing the belief that he was a "police internist" who could cure patients at the state hospital. Even though no recent overtly violent acts were reported, he was committed as needing further inpatient treatment—his medical records revealed that he usually did not respond to therapy in less than four months.

Finally, a word should be said about the role of the family. Surely, if family members wish to testify, this should be allowed, and just as surely, forcing them to do so when they feel unable is unwise. However, some jurisdictions will exclude as hearsay evidence what we have been told by the patient's family (even though we call it history). The relatives may have the only direct evidence of dangerousness, and may, if clinically appropriate, be encouraged to tell it to the judge. It is not easy to testify "against" a relative, even if the clinical staff is convinced that it is in the patient's best interest. A careful balancing of all factors, including the potential reaction of a family member who has testified in favor of commitment only to have the judge release the patient, is in order.

## TREATMENT RIGHTS

The now well-known and broadly accepted concept of a right to treatment for an involuntarily detained psychiatric patient was first introduced by Birnbaum (1960). He spoke of patients in state facilities, commending the staffs and criticizing the legislatures for inadequate appropriations. It was his hope that the courts could enforce this right under the due process clause of the Constitution: treatment would be provided, *quid pro quo,* to justify the temporary deprivation of liberty, and would enable the patient to regain health and freedom with dispatch.

The landmark legal holding that involuntarily committed patients have a constitutionally based right to treatment came in *Wyatt v. Stickney* (1971). The court set forth a series of requirements that were more specific and detailed than most modern-day regulatory requirements. The basic building blocks forming the foundation for adequate treatment have become classic: a humane physical and psychological environment, qualified staff in sufficient numbers, and an individual treatment plan for each patient.

When given the opportunity to do so, the U.S. Supreme Court did not find a right to treatment in the Constitution, but sidestepped the issue (*O'Connor v. Donaldson,* 1975). About as close as that body has come to clarifying treatment rights was in a case involving a very seriously mentally retarded individual in a state facility (*Youngberg v. Romeo,* 1982). There the justices held that due process required reasonably safe conditions of confinement, freedom from unreasonable bodily restraints, and such minimally adequate training as might be required in light of the foregoing rights. The standard set for protection was simply that professional judgment was in fact exercised in coming to a decision.

The convoluted litigation in another right-to-treatment case is detailed elsewhere (Rachlin, 1988). In brief, there have not been radical changes as a result of litigation. However, consent decrees have been signed in lower courts, and the right has found significant favor in state legislatures (Weiner, 1985a). Of course, when executive and legislative branches of state government concur with the judiciary on what needs to be accomplished, important improvements in care can take place. Of further significance is the fact that right-to-treatment issues provide a unique focus of cooperation between clinicians and legal advocates (Appelbaum, 1987).

While useful, the right to treatment is not a panacea. Specifically, it is not a guarantee of treatment for all, nor a right to what might be optimal, nor a means by which the patient can choose his or her own treatment (Appelbaum & Gutheil, 1991).

An outgrowth of the right to treatment is the doctrine that it be provided in the least restrictive alternative. This means, simply, that the government may not pursue its legitimate purposes in ways that broadly stifle personal liberties, or, stated a bit differently, legislative abridgment of rights must utilize the least drastic means of achieving its intended goal. As applied to psychiatry, part of the reason that the least restrictive alternative has found favor is the anti–state-hospital (and pro-community) *zeitgeist* of the 1970s (Miller, 1987).

Clinically applied, to the term "least restrictive alternative" (or environment) must be added the phrase "consistent with the needs of the patient." Thus, for some, a seclusion room is least restrictive because their seriously out-of-control behavior endangers others. By now, the idea of treatment in the least restrictive environment is almost taken for granted, along with the recognition that the environment must include that which is internal to the patient—that is, the illness—as a crucial consideration.

Brief mention needs to be made of other patients' rights. It may be that this is more of an issue in state, as compared with general, hospitals. However, the operative concept is that patients have the same rights as do most other citizens (Weiner, 1985b). For example, patients must be allowed reasonable visitation and other communication, access to attorneys and personal physicians and clergy, and the like. Long lists of particular rights can be found in both legal (Weiner, 1985b; Perlin, 1989) and clinical (Appelbaum & Gutheil, 1991) texts. Before any rights abridgments are undertaken, the clinical reasoning must be carefully thought through and documented in light of the foregoing principles, and must clearly be solely in order to allow treatment to proceed unimpeded. Independent consultation is a useful maneuver when in doubt.

## THE RIGHT TO REFUSE TREATMENT

### Developments in the Law

As recently as a generation ago, nobody knew of any right of a psychiatric patient to refuse pharmacological treatment. When I was a resident, it was considered standard and perfectly acceptable forcibly to inject medication into a patient who was not willing to take it by the oral route.

In the mid-1970s, two federal court cases were instituted in order to establish a right to refuse unwanted treatment. The first of these, in New Jersey, was *Rennie v. Klein* (1978). With concern for the then-current practices in state hospitals, and noting the problem of side effects, the district court judge found a constitutionally based quali-fied right to refuse treatment, except in an emergency. Although the court established a somewhat elaborate scheme for reviewing, and po-tentially overriding, a patient's incompetent refusal, it was built on ex-isting state procedures that called for medical decision making at progressively higher levels within the system and recourse to an inde-pendent psychiatric determination. The limited right to refuse was up-held on appeal, but the review process was simplified. After the case went to the U.S. Supreme Court and was returned to the appellate court for reconsideration in light of *Youngberg v. Romeo* (1982), but without a real decision, the existing scheme again stood affirmed. Thus, through its course, this case held that ultimate decisions relative to refusing patients were to remain in medical hands.

In contrast was the Massachusetts case *Rogers v. Okin* (1979). Soon after this litigation was filed, the district court issued an injunction prohibiting nonconsensual administration of psychopharmacotherapy on several units at Boston State Hospital. Throughout the legal wran-gling here, also based on constitutional arguments, the ultimate deci-sion maker was always a judicially appointed individual. What psychi-atrists consider ordinary treatment for psychosis was labeled by the court as intrusive. Upheld but modified somewhat on initial appeal, *Rogers* got to the U.S. Supreme Court before *Rennie*. The Court re-turned it to the appellate level for reconsideration in light of a state court decision, which held that the guardian of an outpatient could not consent to medication administration (*Guardianship of Roe,* 1981). Although the state's highest court was asked to give its opinion rela-tive to the federal case, and did so, the conclusion was foregone (*Rogers v. Commissioner of Department of Mental Health,* 1983). Only a judge, it was held, could order treatment to be given to an unwilling patient not competent to make his or her own decision. The standard according to which this determination was to be made was a subjective one, substituted judgment. By this is meant that the judge is to ascertain what the patient's desires would be if competent, and to rule in accordance with such a determination.

In New York, the federal courts had approved the state's regulations, which called for clinical review of patients' objections to treatment. Lower state courts agreed. However, in a unanimous (and unexpected) decision, the Court of Appeals held that the state constitution afforded the involuntarily committed patient a fundamental right to refuse antipsychotic medication (*Rivers v. Katz,* 1986). In essence, it was determined here, too, that the state would grant a higher degree of rights protection to its citizens than was required by the U.S. Constitution. In this decision, clinical issues were relegated to a footnote and there was a rather biased litany of the side effects of antipsychotics. The court ruled that a judge must first find the involuntary patient incompetent to make treatment decisions, at a clear and convincing level of proof, and then the judge must determine whether the proposed treatment is "narrowly tailored to give substantive effect to the patient's liberty interest." Here, however, the judge was to use a more objective standard in reaching a decision, that of the best interest of the patient.

Many other states also have gone through right-to-refuse-treatment litigation, with the result in all being the finding of a qualified right to refuse for the involuntary patient. All also have an exception for emergencies, defined differently in the various jurisdictions. Federal courts are no longer a major forum for these cases (Miller, Rachlin, & Appelbaum, 1987). States where there have not been court battles have, by and large, established the substantive right to refuse by legislation or regulation.

Appelbaum (1988) has characterized existing mechanisms for dealing with the procedural aspects of patients' refusals. One set of methods he calls treatment driven: review is in medical hands, either by the treating physician or by an independent review, which can be either internal or external to the institution. The other major division is known as rights driven, and it has three subcategories. In the first, an independent clinician ascertains the patient's competence and the appropriateness of recommended treatment. The second is the situation in which commitment takes place only if the patient is incompetent to make treatment decisions, in essence extinguishing a right to refuse. The third model was discussed in two of the cases outlined above, that is, judicial decision making, occasionally by an appointed guardian, but more likely by a judge.

No clinician can work effectively without knowing and understanding how treatment refusal is dealt with in his or her locale. It bears mention that appellate court decisions tend to underrate the therapeutic benefits of antipsychotics while including long lists of side effects. Trial judges, on the other hand, may be more willing to learn a better balance of the benefits and risks from psychiatrists.

## Research Results

Study of treatment refusal has been a fruitful area for research, with rather consistent outcomes. Appelbaum and Hoge (1986) surveyed both published and unpublished sources and ascertained common results. While a fair number of patients refused medication at some time in their hospital course, far fewer did so persistently. These patients tended to be sicker and more disorganized, with largely illness-based reasons for refusal. Almost all ultimately were treated, with beneficial results, regardless of the method of review. Miller's (1987) analysis of the literature came to basically the same conclusions, and little that has been published subsequently differs materially.

Massachusetts' judicially based system only rarely allowed refusal of medication to stand (Hoge, Gutheil, & Kaplan, 1987). In California, a consent decree calling for independent psychiatric review yielded a 1% rate of denial of authority to medicate, surely not the effect hoped for by the so-called rights advocates (Hargreaves, Shumway, Knutsen, Weinstein, & Senter, 1987). One upstate New York location demonstrated a drop in the number of refusals recorded in the year after the switch from a medical to a judicial model, at both a general and a state hospital, with a significant increase in the number of days to resolution of the disagreement (Ciccone, Tokoli, Clements, & Gift, 1990). However, few changes as a result of the *Rivers* decision were found at a state hospital in New York City (Cournos, McKinnon, & Adams, 1988).

Much important information comes from Hoge et al.'s (1990) prospective study of medication refusal. Most of the patients who rejected treatment in acute-care settings did so within a day or two of admission. They were chronically ill persons who, compared with acceptors, showed significantly greater psychopathology and were less likely to acknowledge their illness. Refusers were hospitalized longer, were more assaultive, and were more likely to be restrained. In those cases that went to court, all patients were approved for involuntary treatment. Of course, in some situations, patients were persuaded to accept medication voluntarily, and a small number were treated without medication.

In most of the foregoing studies, some comment was made about the substantial costs incurred in resolving treatment refusals. Much of this was due to delay in scheduling the court dates for hearings; often a month or more was consumed in the waiting. Schouten and Gutheil (1990) directly assessed costs. For Massachusetts state hospitals alone, over a million dollars was spent per year for additional attorneys and their supporting staffs. Zito, Craig, and Wanderling (1991), in New York, calculated 15,000 potentially avoidable state hospital days annually, because of delays in holding hearings, at an estimated cost of $3.4 million. Why so much time is wasted remains something of a mystery. Courts do not seem impressed by the fact that delaying treatment is, in and of itself, an affirmative decision from a clinical standpoint.

Delays can be especially troublesome in general hospitals. Bloom and colleagues (Bloom, Williams, Goddard, & Faulkner, 1988) report that patients are not being treated in community hospitals if they refuse, thus wasting expensive and valuable days. In an extension of their prior work, Ciccone and colleagues (Ciccone, Tokoli, Gift, & Clements, 1990), again finding no positive patient outcome from treatment refusal, state that insurance benefits from private care may run out while a hearing is pending, and also that attorney fees have to be factored into the hospital's costs. From California, Levin, Brekke, and Thomas (1991) found no judicial upholdings of treatment refusal at an acute-care private university hospital. They, too, document the serious pathology in refusers, the out-of-control behaviors, and other consequences, including increased lengths of stay and necessity for seclusion. Theirs is the only hospital in the county that accepts Medicaid, and they comment that third-party insurers may not reimburse hospitals when treatment does not include an active medication regimen.

Patients in a group studied by Callahan (1986) believed that they should have a qualified right to refuse antipsychotic medication, but they, as forensic patients, may not be representative of the more usual population. Schwartz, Vingiano, and Bezirganian Perez (1988) found that most, but certainly not all, of a series of general hospital patients medicated against their will later agreed that such a maneuver was necessary and important for their treatment.

As pointed out by Simon (1992), all the right-to-refuse-treatment litigation has not, and cannot, provide a meaningful solution to the problem. Some important, but difficult to do, research has not (to my knowledge) yet been performed. I think it crucial to know what happens to involuntarily medicated patients after they leave the hospital. We are all aware that many who voluntarily accept treatment in the hospital fail to comply as outpatients. But if virtually all of those initially unwilling patients then discontinue medication upon discharge, refusal override becomes a very short-term solution indeed.

## Putting Theory into Practice

Perhaps the easiest way for the clinician to view a patient's right to refuse treatment is in the context of the time-honored medicolegal tradition of informed consent. Before someone can be treated, he or she must knowingly, voluntarily, and competently consent to the proposed medical intervention. A voluntary psychiatric patient, one who is virtually by definition competent, thus may not be treated over objection. An involuntary patient is presumed to be competent also, unless evidence exists to demonstrate otherwise. Only in this latter situation would involuntary treatment be possible.

It is not always easy to determine competence. The legal standards fall into one or more of four categories: communicating a choice, understanding relevant information, appreciating the situation and its consequences, or manipulating information rationally (Appelbaum & Grisso, 1988). We all should learn what the law is in our own jurisdictions. But psychiatric patients present special problems. For example, Grisso and Appelbaum (1991) have shown, in a pilot study, that hospitalized schizophrenic patients had generally poorer comprehension of relevant information about pharmacotherapy that is disclosed to them, as compared with depressed, medically ill, and well control groups.

This makes it incumbent on the psychiatrist to work a bit harder to assist patients to understand more fully what they need to know about medications. To the extent that competency means a reasonable understanding of the risks and benefits of, and alternatives (including no treatment) to, a recommended course of therapy, it is a dynamic issue. In bringing this to our attention, Schwartz and Blank (1986) illustrate a situation in which the patient was carefully educated, and, as attention was focused away from a delusional preoccupation, she made a more appropriate assessment of her condition. From his legal perspective, Brooks (1987) suggests that incompetence to make a rational treatment decision requires an incapacity to recognize either the mental illness or the likelihood that medications have beneficial effects.

It should be obvious that the key point is again, as it is relative to civil commitment, that the decisions to be made are clinical. Usual professional skills must be brought to bear before consideration is given to administrative or legal solutions to a patient's refusal of medication. Simon (1992) also believes there has been insufficient appreciation of this dimension.

Even given the fact (see preceding section) that most medication refusals in a general hospital or acute-care setting take place early in the patient's stay, working toward a therapeutic alliance is indicated. Collaboration may be effected thereby (Simon, 1992), and is likely necessary if the patient is to stay on medication for any length of time (Miller, 1987). The clinical effort is justified even when not successful, but at some juncture, a clinical threshold is reached where appropriate measures to attempt to override the treatment refusal are instituted. While this is pending, given the fact that many refusers ultimately agree to accept medication on a voluntary basis, the psychotherapeutic endeavors, any necessary negotiation, and educational work have to continue. Situations such as the nationally publicized B. B. (Billie) Boggs case in New York City, where the hospital discharged this formerly homeless woman, after a lengthy and hard-fought retention, when the judge upheld her right to refuse treatment (see Cournos, 1989), are unfortunate for the profession.

Although not found in early work, psychiatrists must be aware that a proportion of patients who refuse medications do so because of side effects (Callahan, 1986; Hoge et al., 1990). Under these circumstances, one might be hard pressed to demonstrate incompetence, that is, the reason is rational and may not be illness related. Careful clinical assessment and possible modification of the treatment plan by changing medication (or dosage) or adding an anti-Parkinson agent may remedy the problem. Alternatively, the patient may be persuaded that the benefits to be gained in terms of relief of his or her particular symptoms are more important (to the patient) than the discomforting side effects. Tardive dyskinesia is a very real risk over the long term, but not of overarching concern (unless already present) where treatment is measured in terms of a few weeks.

When recourse to a court (or other dispute-resolution mechanism) becomes necessary, my department has found several approaches to be helpful. First, a reasonably wide dosage range is recommended, in order to allow clinical titration without return to court for fine-tuning. Second, a plan for the management of anticipated potential side effects is offered. Finally, we suggest an alternative form of pharmacotherapy, in case the patient does not respond to the first choice. If approval for this package is granted, the patient can be treated as effectively as anyone else on the service. Anecdotally, most patients accept the judge's decision, or require just a few injections before indicating that they would prefer the oral route. As treatment restores competency, patient consent for continuing medication should be obtained.

*Example*

A 29-year-old woman, with a history of several prior hospitalizations and a diagnosis of schizophrenia, paranoid, was admitted after being brought in because of a hostile outburst toward a welfare worker making a home visit. She was overtly psychotic, with Schneiderian first-rank delusions. In the past, she had responded well to pharmacotherapy, but refused such treatment during this hospitalization. A court order to provide medication to her involuntarily was issued after her incompetence was demonstrated by her telling the judge that anybody giving her pills had to be part of a conspiracy.

So where does all of this leave us? Surely a right to refuse treatment is of value to some of the patients some of the time. But what of the risk/benefit ratio, given that only a small percentage of our sickest patients are persistent refusers and that the overwhelming majority of them are ultimately medicated (regardless of the mechanism utilized) after a lot of clinical time, legal system time, and real costs, resulting from these factors plus extended hospitalization and treatment (read symptom relief) are delayed? In the past, I suppose I have approved involuntary treatment for an occasional possibly competent refuser, and I know that I used to look at the issues as being as much administrative in nature as clinical. Perhaps, then, Brooks (1987) is correct in pointing out that the heuristic value of refusal litigation is a major accomplishment that is not to be underestimated. As I have concluded elsewhere (Rachlin, 1989), the right to appropriate and thoughtful treatment is what the best interest of the patient is really about.

## REFERENCES

*Addington v. Texas,* 441 U.S. 418, 99 S.Ct. 1804 (1979).

Appelbaum, P. S. (1987). Resurrecting the right to treatment. *Hospital and Community Psychiatry, 38,* 703–704, 721.

Appelbaum, P. S. (1988). The right to refuse treatment with antipsychotic medications: Retrospect and prospect. *American Journal of Psychiatry, 145,* 413–419.

Appelbaum, P. S., & Grisso, T. (1988). Assessing patients' capacities to consent to treatment. *New England Journal of Medicine, 319,* 1635–1638.

Appelbaum, P. S., & Gutheil, T. G. (1991). *Clinical handbook of psychiatry and the law* (2d ed.). Baltimore, MD: Williams & Wilkins.

Appelbaum, P. S., & Hoge, S. K. (1986). The right to refuse treatment: What the research reveals. *Behavioral Sciences and the Law, 4,* 279–292.

Bagby, R. M., Thompson, J. S., Dickens, S. E., & Nohara, M. (1991). Decision making in psychiatric civil commitment: An experimental analysis. *American Journal of Psychiatry, 148,* 28–33.

Birnbaum, M. (1960). The right to treatment. *American Bar Association Journal, 46,* 499–505.

Bloom, J. D., Williams, M. H., Goddard, S. L., & Faulkner, L. R. (1988). The influence of the right to refuse treatment on precommitment patients. *Bulletin of the American Academy of Psychiatry and the Law, 16,* 5–9.

Brooks, A. D. (1987). The right to refuse antipsychotic medications: Law and policy. *Rutgers Law Review, 39,* 339–376.

Bursztajn, H., Gutheil, T. G., Hamm, R. M., Brodsky, A., & Mills, M. J. (1988). *Parens patriae* considerations in the commitment process. *Psychiatric Quarterly, 59,* 165–181.

Bursztajn, H., Gutheil, T. G., Mills, M., Hamm, R. M., & Brodsky, A. (1986). Process analysis of judges' commitment decisions: A preliminary empirical study. *American Journal of Psychiatry, 143,* 170–174.

Callahan, L. A. (1986). Changing mental health law: Butting heads with a billygoat. *Behavioral Sciences and the Law, 4,* 305–314.

Ciccone, J. R., Tokoli, J. F., Clements, C. D., & Gift, T. E. (1990). Right to refuse treatment: Impact of *Rivers v. Katz. Bulletin of the American Academy of Psychiatry and the Law, 18,* 203–215.

Ciccone, J. R., Tokoli, J. J., Gift, T. E., & Clements, C. D. (1990). Treatment refusal and judicial activism: A re-examination. Presented at the 143rd Annual Meeting of the American Psychiatric Association, New York City, May.

Cleveland, S., Mulvey, E. P., Appelbaum, P. S., & Lidz, C. W. (1989). Do dangerousness-oriented commitment laws restrict hospitalization of patients who need treatment? A test. *Hospital and Community Psychiatry, 40,* 266–271.

Cournos, F. (1989). Involuntary medication and the case of Joyce Brown. *Hospital and Community Psychiatry, 40,* 736–740.

Cournos, F., McKinnon, K., & Adams, C. (1988). A comparison of clinical and judicial procedures for reviewing requests for involuntary medication in New York. *Hospital and Community Psychiatry, 39,* 851–855.

Durham, M. L., & LaFond, J. Q. (1985). The empirical consequences and policy implications of broadening the statutory criteria for civil commitment. *Yale Law and Policy Review, 3,* 395–446.

*Guardianship of Roe,* 383 Mass. 415, 421 N.E.2d 40 (1981).

Grisso, T., & Appelbaum, P. S. (1991). Mentally ill and non-mentally ill patients' abilities to understand informed consent disclosures for medication: Preliminary data. *Law and Human Behavior, 15,* 377–388.

Gutheil, T. G., Rachlin, S., & Mills, M. J. (1985). Differing conceptual models in psychiatry and law. *New Directions for Mental Health Services No. 25,* 5–11.

Hargreaves, W. A., Shumway, M., Knutsen, E. J., Weinstein, A., & Senter, N. (1987). Effects of the *Jamison-Farabee* consent decree: Due process protection for involuntary psychiatric patients treated with psychoactive medication. *American Journal of Psychiatry, 144,* 188–192.

Hiday, V. A., & Smith, L. N. (1987). Effects of the dangerousness standard in civil commitment. *Journal of Psychiatry and Law, 15,* 433–454.

Hoge, S. K., Appelbaum, P. S., & Geller, J. L. (1989). Involuntary treatment. In A. Tasman, R. E. Hales, & A. J. Frances (Eds.), *Review of psychiatry* (Vol. 8, pp. 432–450). Washington, DC: American Psychiatric Press.

Hoge, S. K., Appelbaum, P. S., & Greer, A. (1989). An empirical comparison of the Stone and dangerousness criteria for civil commitment. *American Journal of Psychiatry, 146,* 170–175.

Hoge, S. K., Appelbaum, P. S., Lawlor, T., Beck, J. C., Litman, R., Greer, A., Gutheil, T. G., & Kaplan, E. (1990). A prospective, multicenter study of patients' refusal of antipsychotic medication. *Archives of General Psychiatry, 47,* 949–956.

Hoge, S. K., Gutheil, T. G., & Kaplan, E. (1987). The right to refuse treatment under *Rogers v. Commissioner:* Preliminary empirical findings and comparisons. *Bulletin of the American Academy of Psychiatry and the Law, 15,* 163–169.

Hoge, S. K., Sachs, G., Appelbaum, P. S., Greer, A., & Gordon, C. (1988). Limitations on psychiatrists' discretionary civil commitment authority by the Stone and dangerousness criteria. *Archives of General Psychiatry, 45,* 764–769.

*Jones v. United States,* 463 U.S. 354, 103 S.Ct. 3043 (1983).

Levin, S., Brekke, J. S., & Thomas, P. (1991). A controlled comparison of involuntarily hospitalized medication refusers and acceptors. *Bulletin of the American Academy of Psychiatry and the Law, 19,* 161–171.

Lidz, C. W., Mulvey, E. P., Appelbaum, P. S., & Cleveland, S. (1989). Commitment: The consistency of clinicians and the use of legal standards. *American Journal of Psychiatry, 146,* 176–181.

McFarland, B. H., Faulkner, L. R., Bloom, J. D., Hallaux, R. J., & Bray, J. D. (1989). Investigators' and judges' opinions about civil commitment. *Bulletin of the American Academy of Psychiatry and the Law, 17,* 15–24.

Miller, R. D. (1985). Involuntary civil commitment: Legal versus clinical paternalism. *New Directions for Mental Health Services No. 25,* 13–24.

Miller, R. D. (1987). *Involuntary civil commitment of the mentally ill in the post-reform era.* Springfield, IL: Charles C. Thomas.

Miller, R. D. (1990). Involuntary civil commitment. In R. I. Simon (Ed.), *Review of clinical psychiatry and the law* (Vol. 2, pp. 95–172). Washington, DC: American Psychiatric Press.

Miller, R. D., Maier, G. J., & Kaye, M. (1985). *Miranda* comes to the hospital: The right to remain silent in civil commitment. *American Journal of Psychiatry, 142,* 1074–1077.

Miller, R. D., Rachlin, S., & Appelbaum, P. S. (1987). Patients' rights: The action moves to state courts. *Hospital and Community Psychiatry, 38,* 343–344.

*O'Connor v. Donaldson*, 422 U.S. 563, 95 S.Ct. 2486 (1975).

Perlin, M. L. (1989). *Mental disability law: Civil and criminal* (vols. 1–3). Charlottesville, VA: Michie.

Rachlin, S. (1983). The influence of law on deinstitutionalization. *New Directions for Mental Health Services No. 17*, 41–54.

Rachlin, S. (1987). Redefining dangerousness for civil commitment. *Hospital and Community Psychiatry, 38*, 884–886.

Rachlin, S. (1988). Litigating a right to treatment: *Woe* is me. *Psychiatric Quarterly, 59*, 182–192.

Rachlin, S. (1989). Rethinking the right to refuse treatment. *Psychiatric Annals, 19*, 213–222.

*Rennie v. Klein*, 462 F.Supp. 1131 (D.N.J. 1978), *suppl.*, 476 F.Supp. 1294 (D.N.J. 1979), *modified*, 653 F.2d 836 (3d Cir. 1981), *vacated and remanded*, 458 U.S. 1119, 102 S.Ct. 3506 (1982), *on remand*, 720 F.2d 266 (3d Cir. 1983).

*Rivers v. Katz*, 67 N.Y.2d 485, 495 N.E.2d 337 (1986).

*Rogers v. Com'r of Dept. of Mental Health*, 390 Mass. 489, 458 N.E.2d 308 (1983).

*Rogers v. Okin*, 478 F.Supp. 1342 (D.Mass. 1979), *modified*, 634 F.2d 650 (1st Cir. 1980), *vacated and remanded*, 457 U.S. 291, 102 S.Ct. 2442 (1982), *on remand*, 738 F.2d 1 (1st Cir. 1984).

Schouten, R., & Gutheil, T. G. (1990). Aftermath of the *Rogers* decision: Assessing the costs. *American Journal of Psychiatry, 147*, 1348–1352.

Schwartz, H. I., Appelbaum, P. S., & Kaplan, R. D. (1984). Clinical judgments in the decision to commit. *Archives of General Psychiatry, 41*, 811–815.

Schwartz, H. I., & Blank, K. (1986). Shifting competency during hospitalization: A model for informed consent decisions. *Hospital and Community Psychiatry, 37*, 1256–1260.

Schwartz, H. I., Vingiano, W., & Bezirganian Perez, C. (1988). Autonomy and the right to refuse treatment: Patients' attitudes after involuntary medication. *Hospital and Community Psychiatry, 39*, 1049–1054.

Segal, S. P., Watson, M. A., Goldfinger, S. M., & Averbuck, D. S. (1988). Civil commitment in the psychiatric emergency room: II. Mental disorder indicators and three dangerousness criteria. *Archives of General Psychiatry, 45*, 753–758.

Simon, R. I. (1992). *Clinical psychiatry and the law.* (2d ed.) Washington, DC: American Psychiatric Press.

Stromberg, C. D., & Stone, A. A. (1983). A model state law on civil commitment of the mentally ill. *Harvard Journal on Legislation, 20*, 275–396.

Weiner, B. A. (1985a). Treatment rights. In S. J. Brakel, J. Parry, & B. A. Weiner (Eds.). *The mentally disabled and the law* (3d ed.) (pp. 327–367). Chicago, IL: American Bar Foundation.

Weiner, B. A. (1985b). Rights of institutionalized persons. In S. J. Brakel, J. Parry, & B. A. Weiner (Eds.). *The mentally disabled and the law* (3d ed.) (pp. 251–325). Chicago, IL: American Bar Foundation.

*Wyatt v. Stickney,* 325 F.Supp. 781 (M.D.Ala. 1971), 334 F.Supp. 1341 (M.D. Ala. 1971), *enforced,* 344 F.Supp. 373 (M.D. Ala. 1972), 344 F.Supp. 387 (M.D. Ala. 1972), *aff'd in part sub nom. Wyatt v. Aderholt,* 503 F.2d 1305 (5th Cir. 1974).

*Youngberg v. Romeo,* 457 U.S. 307, 102 S.Ct. 2452 (1982).

Zito, J. M., Craig, T. J., & Wanderling, J. (1991). New York under the *Rivers* decision: An epidemiologic study of drug treatment refusal. *American Journal of Psychiatry, 148,* 904–909.

# 5

# Management of Assaultive Patients on the Psychiatric Unit of the General Hospital
## Legal and Ethical Considerations

The management of assaultive patients on the psychiatric unit of the general hospital poses enormous challenges to clinicians. Of course, clinicians have always been concerned about assaults by patients. In recent years, however, their concern has intensified because the problem of violence on psychiatric wards appears to have worsened, while the legal regulations governing the management of violent patients have become increasingly complex.

Because different hospitals use different criteria to define and document violent behavior, and nurses and other staff members generally report only the most serious incidents, valid data on rates of inpatient violence are difficult to obtain. Nonetheless, a number of authors have suggested that rates of assault by psychiatric inpatients have been increasing (Adler, Kreeger, & Ziegler, 1983; Haller & Deluty, 1988; Rossi et al., 1985). On the other hand, Reid, Bolinger, and Edwards (1989), in a major survey of assaults by patients in hospitals, found a relatively small rate of assaults (1.36 assaults per bed per year) on adult psychiatric units, and found that only nine (5.7%) of 158 reported assault victims required medical treatment. But even Reid and co-workers concede that their findings of low rates and severity of assaults may not reflect actual dangerousness in hospitals because of hospitals' varying safety policies concerning coping with dangerous patients and protecting staff and other patients.

Significantly, many researchers report high percentages of patients who have been assaultive prior to admission; such patients have ranged in the various studies from 11% to 15% (Binder & McNeil, 1986; Craig, 1982; Travin & Bluestone, 1987). Even more striking are the findings of Rofman, Askinazi, and Fant (1980) that 24 (41%) of 59 patients committed on an emergency basis to a Veterans Administration Hospital for dangerousness to others had engaged in assaultive behavior after admission, the greatest frequency of these assaults occurring within the first 10 days of hospitalization. Similarly, McNeil and Binder (1987) also reported that more than two-thirds of patients civilly committed for dangerousness to others engaged in some form of violent behavior, including dangerous activities, verbal assaults, and physical assaults, within the first 72 hours of hospitalization.

With a convergence of a variety of factors, including the dangerousness criterion for involuntary admission, the deinstitutionalization that resulted in increased numbers of severely mentally ill patients seeking treatment in local hospitals, the patients' right to refuse medication resulting in delays in stabilizing aggressive patients, increased numbers of impulsive and/or character-disordered patients, and the general reluctance to discharge violence-prone patients back to the community, psychiatric units, especially those in urban areas, are likely to contain a greater percentage of dangerous patients than in previous years. It is, therefore, necessary for clinicians practicing in psychiatric units to acquire state-of-the-art skills and knowledge with regard to the management of violent patients. Clinicians also need to be aware of existing statutes, regulations, and their own hospital guidelines or procedures for medicating patients against their will, employing seclusion and restraint, administratively discharging character-disordered patients, determining the appropriateness of prosecution of assaultive patients, and discharging compensated but potentially violent psychiatric inpatients. Clearly, decision making in the management of violent patients involves negotiating and resolving myriad and complicated psychiatric–legal issues.

## MULTIPLE FACTORS IN THE PREDICTION
## OF POTENTIAL VIOLENCE

Clinicians' ability to predict potential violence in psychiatric inpatients so as to take preventive measures would be enhanced if valid correlates of violent behavior could be identified. While the accuracy of clinicians' long-term predictions of violence by patients released from institutions has been discredited, their short-term predictive capabilities seem to be more promising. Accordingly, predictive research has been focusing on determining the various factors that appear to increase the short-term risk of inpatient violence.

Increasingly, violence has been described as resulting from multiple factors (Tupin, 1983). Brizer (1989) reviews a variety of factors reported to be correlates of violent behavior, grouping them into trait predictors, state predictors, and situational variables (p. XIII). Under the rubric "trait predictors," Brizer briefly discusses the likelihood of an association between violence and such variables as (younger) age, (male) gender, legal status of dangerousness, and history of violent behavior. Under the rubric "state predictors," Brizer points out that patients' shifting cognitive and physiological states are at least as important as determinants of violent behavior as are patients' more permanent characteristics, such as race and gender. Although many researchers have reported an association between the diagnosis of schizophrenia and inpatient violence, the question of whether patients having certain psychiatric diagnoses are particularly at risk for violent behavior is still far from resolved. Under the title "situational variables," Brizer outlines such situational and interactional factors as time of day, overcrowding, behavior of the victim, the staff, and countertransference issues.

Based on studies conducted in an intensive-psychiatric-care unit of a Veterans Administration Center, Yesavage and Brizer (1989) describe the major correlates of dangerous behavior in this patient sample as severe psychosis, low neuroleptic blood levels, severity of violent behavior before admission, military combat experience, and childhood discipline. Other potential correlates considered were race, drug abuse, and self-destructive behavior. In a review article on violence by psychiatric inpatients, Davis (1991) emphasizes that an overall model of violence must include such individual factors as diagnosis, stage of illness, behavior, and cognition; such situational factors as the physical environment of the ward and the various staff members and other patients; and such structural factors as restrictive commitment and detention policies, a shortage of beds, and inadequate community resources, resulting in more seriously disturbed and personality-disordered patients being treated on psychiatric units.

## IMMINENT VIOLENCE AND
## EMERGENCY INTERVENTION

The rapid assessment of imminent violence and the choice of appropriate clinical intervention to prevent it constitute a true emergency. In this situation, the clinician must assess the patient's behavioral cues of posture, speech, motor activity, and startle response (Dubin & Stolberg, 1981). Hanke (1984) emphasizes that the patient's escalating psychomotor activity and extreme affect may indicate an impending loss of control of his or her hostile impulses. Lee and colleagues (Lee, Villar, Juthani, & Bluestone, 1989) found that the majority of patients who had engaged in reported incidents of physical violence on an acute-care psychiatric ward had been hyperactive, verbally abusive, loud, angry, or hostile immediately before the incidents, which suggests that behavior patterns might have better predictive value than diagnosis. Based on the assessment, the clinician must decide whether the threat of violence is serious enough to justify emergency intervention. The clinician may be guided in this decision by his or her experience with the patient's previous pattern of behavior that resulted in assaultive behavior.

As Appelbaum (1987) points out, the clinician's decision requires his or her balancing of two sets of patients' rights—the right to be free of unnecessary restraint and the right to be free of violent assault. The U.S. Supreme Court decision in *Youngberg v. Romeo* (1982) recognized this conflict by holding that the patient's protected liberty rights under the Due Process Clause of the Fourteenth Amendment had to be balanced against relevant state reasons for restraining individual liberty. The professional can achieve this balance by making a competent decision that does not substantially depart from accepted professional judgment, practice, and standards. Clinicians are thereby accorded professional discretion, within the parameters of competent practice and standards of care, in deciding the degree of restrictions needed to protect both the patient and others from assault. Appelbaum (1987) emphasizes that, for a variety of ethical, clinical, and legal reasons, in making decisions about potential violence, it is better to decide temporarily to restrict the patient's freedom of movement in order to prevent assault than to respect the patient's freedom to the extent of allowing an assault to occur.

Depending on the situation, the clinician decides among several courses of intervention: verbal, medication, physical (seclusion and restraint), or some combination of these measures. Clearly, the least restrictive of these measures is verbal intervention, which often results in the patient's agreeing to take an increased amount of medication to help calm him or her down and to restore his or her control. If this treatment approach fails or is inappropriate, the clinician must take more restrictive measures. Wexler (1984) notes that there has been some disagreement about the relative restrictiveness of forced medication as compared with physical restraint and seclusion. For example, Dix (1987) argues that physical restraint is the least restrictive alternative, while Soloff (1987) would employ physical controls for violent behavior not responding to verbal or chemical intervention. Although *Youngberg v. Romeo* did not explicitly discuss the "least restrictive" doctrine, Wexler notes that the Court's statement that "it is not appropriate for the courts to specify which of several professionally acceptable choices should have been made" (p. 2461) may discourage courts from constructing a ranking order of restrictiveness among the various methods of seclusion and restraint. Certainly, clinicians must exercise their best clinical judgment in employing one or a combination of intervention techniques most suitable for the needs of the patient.

## EMERGENCY INVOLUNTARY MEDICATION

Although clinicians' discretion concerning the use of medication for patients who refuse treatment has been legally restricted to protect patients' liberty and privacy rights, clinicians are permitted to administer medication against a patient's will in an emergency situation. While the definition of "emergency" has varied somewhat in different jurisdictions, medication to prevent imminent physical assault that could result in injury would be permitted in all jurisdictions. Tardiff (1991) emphasizes that emergency medication can be used instead of seclusion or restraint, or in combination with seclusion or restraint in a severely agitated or violent psychotic patient, and that neuroleptic medication should be used principally for violent patients with psychotic symptoms. Tardiff also points out that lawsuits pertaining to excessive seclusion or restraint or to injuries occurring in seclusion or on the psychiatric ward can raise questions about whether the right medications and dosages were used, and that patients should not be kept in seclusion or restraint for excessive periods because of inadequate medication. Consequently, it is important for clinicians to be knowledgeable about psychopharmacology, including the indications for rapid neuroleptization either by a high-potency neuroleptic combined with an anxiolytic or sedating drug such as intramuscular haloperidol (Haldol) and lorazepam (Ativan), or by a low-potency neuroleptic such as chlorpromazine (Thorazine), which has both antipsychotic and sedative effects.

Appelbaum (1983) underscores the distinction between the use of antipsychotic medication for immediate sedative effects to manage patients in emergencies (the use of which, in such cases, would be subject to the legal controls of restraining patients) and the increase of antipsychotic medication following an assault, in which case the medication would be subject to the same legal regulations as for the treatment of nonviolent patients. Because the courts are sensitive to the possibility that medication might be used for sedation rather than for treatment, Appelbaum recommends that antipsychotics should not be used strictly for sedation. However, if the patient requires both sedation and antipsychotic treatment, an antipsychotic agent is the preferred medication.

### Case 1: Medication and Seclusion

Mr. A., a 23-year-old single man, was readmitted to the psychiatric unit because of paranoid fears and his threatening his mother with violence. He had been hospitalized previously for acute psychosis, was diagnosed as paranoid schizophrenic, and after having engaged in several assaults on the ward, eventually was successfully treated with antipsychotic medication.

Upon this present admission to the ward, Mr. A. agreed to take the prescribed antipsychotic medication, which seemed to calm him down and reduce the intensity of his paranoid fears. After several days, however, he adamantly refused to take any more medication, claiming that the "doctors were drugging" him and that he was becoming "too slow to fight" his enemies. While the necessary procedures were being followed to take the case to court in order to obtain permission to medicate the patient against his will, Mr. A.'s agitated and paranoid behavior began to escalate. During one lunch hour, he angrily accused the staff of planning to kill him and began pacing up and down the ward, bumping into other patients, shouting obscenities, and threatening staff members. All attempts to talk to him were met with increased agitation, paranoid accusations, and threats of violence.

The psychiatrist evaluated the situation, determined that the patient was at serious risk for assault, and ordered an intramuscular injection of medication over the patient's refusal. Despite the intramuscular medication, Mr. A. continued to make threatening remarks and gestures, so the staff escorted him into the seclusion room. The patient stayed in the seclusion room for approximately one and a half hours, and then, after being deemed to be calmer and no longer imminently violent, was released from seclusion. During the next two days, the patient had two more such episodes of marked agitation and threats of violence, though he calmed down considerably after being administered involuntary medication and did not have to be confined in the seclusion room. By the third day, Mr. A. consented to resume taking his prescribed oral medication, and his mental condition steadily improved.

*Discussion of Case 1*

The basic psychiatric–legal decisions in this case were the determination of imminent violence and the choice of intervention modality[ies] needed to manage this psychotic violent patient. Clearly, clinicians must carefully assess the likelihood of an assault occurring before using any involuntary treatment modality. Based on the patient's prior history of assaults, and on his acute psychotic state with marked agitation, hostility, loudness, and threatening behavior, the psychiatrist determined that this was an emergency situation requiring immediate intervention. Since talking to the patient proved useless, the psychiatrist initially chose involuntary medication. Acting on the psychiatrist's orders, the staff temporarily restrained the patient and administered the injection. In choosing this treatment, the psychiatrist had to consider both the correct medication and a dosage adequate to sedate but not enough to "snow" the patient and cause him to fall asleep or become groggy, in a kind of "chemical seclusion" (Appleton, 1965, p. 92).

An antipsychotic was the choice of emergency medication because of the patient's acute paranoid psychosis. Because the patient remained agitated and continued to make threatening gestures, the staff decided to place him in the seclusion room. It is important to note that the psychiatrist did not order medication on an as-needed basis (p.r.n.: *pro re nata*), but instead ordered a fixed dose regimen and directed that he be immediately summoned to reevaluate the patient if any changes in his condition occurred. It is also important to point out that the neuroleptic medication administered intramuscularly consisted of single injections sufficient only to control the emergency situation, despite the patient's remaining psychotic and thus offering a strong possibility of a return of the violent behavior.

Appelbaum and Gutheil (1991) comment that this restriction on the scope of medication is consistent with a "nonclinical" view that medication is chiefly for the purpose of controlling behavior, rather than for the treatment of mental illness. But even under a strict definition of emergency, with the inherent uncertainty of when an emergency begins and at what moment to initiate involuntary medication, Appelbaum and Gutheil believe that a repetitively assaultive patient with a known pattern of building up to a physical attack need not be allowed to assault someone before medication may be administered. In the case discussed, after receiving intramuscular medication after each of the next two violence-threatening episodes, Mr. A. calmed down and ceased making any threatening remarks or gestures, so the staff did not deem it necessary to confine him in the seclusion room. Interestingly, Mr. A. ultimately consented to take oral medication before the case for administering medication against his will could be decided in the courtroom.

## SECLUSION AND RESTRAINT

Although the use of seclusion and restraint may seem to some nonclinicians to be obsolete relics of past psychiatric treatment, in actuality, these modalities of emergency interventions are vital parts of the armamentarium in the contemporary management of violent psychiatric inpatients. The *Rogers v. Okin* (1979) case in Massachusetts focused a great deal of attention on the subject when the court explicitly ruled that the use of seclusion be restricted to "emergency situations in which there was occurrence of serious threat of extreme violence, personal injury, or attempted suicide" (p. 1343). While the Supreme Court in the *Youngberg v. Romeo* case in 1982 deferred to the professional's judgment in deciding the necessity for restraining individual liberty in emergency situations, it is important for clinicians to be aware that some jurisdictions have more rigorous state statutes and regulations than are needed to satisfy *Romeo*'s constitutional safeguards (Tardiff, 1984). Consequently, clinicians should be aware of the legal limitations imposed in the states in which they practice.

With regard to formulating a specific policy on seclusion and restraint, Tardiff (1984) believes that this should be addressed through the more pliable mechanism of hospital policy and administrative regulations, rather than through rigid legislation. The Joint Commission on Accreditation of Health Care Organizations (JCAHO) requires hospitals to develop written policies and procedures for the use of special treatment procedures that require justification, such as restraint and seclusion, and to ensure documentation of the use of these procedures in medical records. A violation of hospital policy and an injury to the patient would be legally indefensible (Simon, 1987). Halleck (1980) warns that, in general, psychiatric hospitals are liable for battery when patients are physically abused by staff. Also, it is not inconceivable that, if a physician becomes involved in physically restraining a patient in an excessively forceful manner, the physician, as well as the hospital, could be sued for assault and battery.

In a review of 13 studies on seclusion and restraint in adult inpatient psychiatric settings, Soloff, Gutheil, and Wexler (1985) found that there was a great deal of variation in the findings. The incidence rate of seclusion varied, for example, from a low of 1.9% in a chronic state hospital (Tardiff, 1981), through a rate of 26% at a university municipal hospital in New York City (Plutchik, Karasu, Conte, Siegel, & Jerrett, 1978), to a rate of 44% in a short-term crisis intervention unit (Binder, 1979), and finally to a high of 66% in a research unit for schizophrenia that was medication-free (Wadeson & Carpenter, 1976).

Thus the incidence of seclusion seemed to vary mostly with the patient population served and the treatment philosophy of the ward. In general, schizophrenic and manic patients seemed to be at highest risk for seclusion in acute-care settings. Regarding the precipitating events that led to the use of seclusion, nine of the reported studies attributed the greatest use of seclusion to a pattern of disruptive behavior described as "agitated, uncontrolled behavior" and "escalating agitation" (Soloff et al., 1985, p. 656). As for patients' reactions to the seclusion experience, different studies reported varying feelings about the experience. Soloff et al. concluded that seclusion is rarely used for punitive purposes or merely to attain custodial control, and that there is overwhelming empirical support for using seclusion and restraint to contain the progressive deterioration of disruptive behavior to actual violence.

In 1984, the American Psychiatric Association (APA) published extensive guidelines in this important area, titled *The Psychiatric Uses of Seclusion and Restraint,* edited by Kenneth Tardiff, M.D. In this volume, Gutheil and Tardiff (1984) outline some of the indications for and contraindications to seclusion and restraint from a clinical model of exercising reasonable clinical judgment rather than from a legal model with its strict reliance on regulations, procedures, and statutes. In this clinical model, the main indications for seclusion and restraint would be to prevent imminent harm to the patient or others, to prevent a serious disruption of the treatment program, to assist the treatment as part of an ongoing behavioral therapy, to decrease the stimulation a patient receives, and to comply with a patient's request. Gutheil and Tardiff underscore as a major clinical contraindication to seclusion a patient's unstable medical condition, such as cardiac illness or metabolic illness, that requires close monitoring, though restraint in such cases may be of value. Other relative contraindications to seclusion include a patient's paradoxical reaction to phenothiazine medication and symptoms of uncontrollable self-abuse and self-mutilation. Serious adverse effects of physical restraint are circulatory obstruction, which staff members must deal with by alternately releasing one of four-point restraints every 15 minutes, and the possibility of aspiration, which they must prevent by constant monitoring. Placing patients in seclusion for punitive reasons or for staff comfort and convenience is absolutely contraindicated. Other misuses of seclusion include leaving the patient for long periods without adequate checking and monitoring, possibly constituting a form of abandonment; seclusion as a form of scapegoating a particular patient; and seclusion as a nonconstructive reaction to a patient's provocative or attention-seeking behavior.

With regard to the implementation of seclusion and restraint, Lion and Soloff (1984) outline the procedure as being initiated in general by nursing and other professional staff members in compliance with hospital policy. Briefly, the staff should notify the physician as soon as possible, preferably within one hour, and, for the first episode, the physician should see the patient usually within three hours, and preferably within one hour, after initiation of the procedure. The physician should examine the patient carefully, review the order for seclusion or restraint, and document in the patient's record the need for its continuation. The physician should indicate any special precautions and monitoring that must be undertaken by the nursing and other professional staff. And he or she should see the patient as often as deemed necessary, with a minimum of two visits a day, at 12-hour intervals. Nursing staff should observe the patient's behavior every 15 minutes.

Clinicians are advised to review the APA's guidelines on seclusion and restraint in order to gain more detailed knowledge on such crucial topics as initiation and review, physician monitoring, general comments about restraint and seclusion maneuvers, specific techniques, care of the patient and staff, and removal of the patient from seclusion and restraint. As Lion and Soloff underscore, seclusion and restraint techniques are as important in scope as are the medical procedures of cardio-pulmonary resuscitation (CPR), and should be in the armamentarium of any psychiatric facility.

## Case 2: Seclusion and Restraint

Mr. B., a 31-year-old homeless and chronically mentally ill man, was admitted to the psychiatric unit on emergency status because of marked agitation, paranoid delusions, and bizarre behavior. He had been found in the street, wandering aimlessly and directing traffic.

A mental-status examination revealed him to be suspicious, guarded, and mildly agitated, and as having a thought disorder with derailment and illogical responses and a paranoid delusion that drug enforcement agents wanted to kill him because he had once worked for them as an undercover agent. He acknowledged that he had been a patient in several state hospitals and had received a variety of medications, but flatly refused to grant permission to the staff to contact these hospitals. He did agree to take a small oral dose of a high-potency neuroleptic medication, which he agreed had once helped him in the past.

Initially, he seemed to be improving; he appeared calmer and participated in ward activities. Suddenly, on the fourth day in the day room, he became markedly agitated and, without any provocation, began to accuse another patient of planning to attack him; before the staff could intervene, he punched the patient. He then threw a chair at the wall and shouted that everybody was involved in the plot against him. He threatened to defend himself and to strike anybody who came near him. The other patients were escorted out of the area, the security guards were summoned, and the staff members restrained and escorted Mr. B. into the seclusion room, where he was administered emergency medication despite his protests that he would no longer take any medication. In the seclusion room, Mr. B. began punching the wall with his fists. He was immediately taken out and put into sheet restraints and kept under constant observation. The staff contacted the state hospital at which he had most recently been a patient and learned that it had had a similar experience with him, that he had to be kept in physical restraints on several occasions, and that the medication that finally helped him was a substantial dose of a low-potency neuroleptic medication. This information proved to be quite important in the further management of this patient.

## Discussion of Case 2

Among the emergencies that clinicians working in an inpatient unit must deal with immediately and decisively are outbursts of violence, which often take place suddenly and without provocation or warning. Clinicians must protect the other patients and staff, as well as the violent patient himself or herself, from harm. As this case illustrates, the other patients were escorted to safety, the security guards were summoned as a show of force and to be available to assist if needed, and the patient's out-of-control behavior was dealt with in accordance with hospital policy, which follows state laws and regulations. In New York, restraint and seclusion can be used "only when absolutely necessary to protect the patient from injuring himself or herself or others" (New

York Official Compilation, 1986). And the New York Mental Hygiene Law specifies that restraints, meaning an apparatus that prevents free movement, should be employed only if less restrictive techniques have been determined to be inadequate to avoid injury, that the "camisole" and the "full or partial restraining sheet" or other less restrictive restraints are the only forms of permissible restraint, and that restraints should be implemented only by written order of a physician after a personal examination. But if a physician is not immediately available, restraint may be employed only to an extent needed to prevent injury, and pending the arrival of the physician, the patient should be kept under constant observation. The physician must respond within 30 minutes. The patient's condition is assessed at least every 30 minutes. (This hospital's policy is to document on the restraint record every 15 minutes by the nursing staff and every two hours at a minimum by the registered nurse.) At least every two hours, the patient is released from restraint, and if there are no overt gestures that threaten serious harm or injury, the restraints should not be reimposed and the physician is to be notified immediately (New York Mental Hygiene Law, 1988).

Another important psychiatric–legal determination in this case was the question of breach of confidentiality. While the staff did not initially contact the state hospital where the patient was last treated, in the emergent situation created by the patient's violent behavior, staff members telephoned that facility and were able to obtain crucial information about the management of the patient.

## ADMINISTRATIVE DISCHARGE OF THE ASSAULTIVE INPATIENT

As Appelbaum and Gutheil (1991) emphasize, inpatient clinicians have dual responsibilities—to both the individual patient and to others on the ward. Thus clinicians faced with a dangerous patient must assess the patient's "differential dangerousness" on the ward or off of it in their determinations on whether the patient can be involuntarily discharged (p. 125). Among the factors clinicians must consider are the patient's committability, psychotic state, treatability, and degree of dangerousness to other patients. Appelbaum and Gutheil point out that involuntary discharge for dangerousness is actually in the patient's best interests, because the patient's further stay on the ward may result in his or her increased anxiety, guilt, or criminal charges resulting from continued assaultiveness. While pressing charges may have some value in personality-disordered patients as an external limit-setting maneuver, in cases of severely mentally ill patients, the criminal justice system is generally reluctant to pursue prosecution.

Although prosecution is rarely initiated against patients who have assaulted others on the psychiatric ward, the determining factors in deciding this matter have come under increased discussion in recent years. Phelan, Mills, and Ryan (1985) reported the case of a nurse who was physically attacked and almost throttled by a man with a history of severe depression on an inpatient ward, and who decided, with much ambivalence, to press charges against him. Phelan et al. believe that the decision to press charges raises a variety of ethical questions and conflicting concerns, but suggest that professionals may have a duty to do so in cases of serious assault, not only to make the assault part of the public record and to allow a judge or jury to attribute responsibility, but also because initiating prosecution should lead to a diminution of violent acts by other patients who may be able to exercise control over themselves. Joining the debate on this issue, Gutheil (1985) asserts that any litigation would tend irrevocably to undermine the therapeutic alliance, and perhaps inspire responses from the patient regarding the clinician's use of emergency physical restraints; that no research supports the idea that knowledge of possible prosecution tends to diminish assaults by patients; and that it is erroneous to suggest that professionals may have a duty to initiate charges, as no such duty has ever been defined. Miller and Maier (1987), on the other hand, point out that with the growing number of personality-disordered and chronically aggressive patients being treated in civil hospitals, the option of initiating criminal charges should at least be available to staff members for purposes of morale.

## Case 3: Discharging the Violent Patient

Mr. C., a 29-year-old single, unemployed man residing with his sister and brother-in-law, was brought into the emergency room by his sister. She reported that her brother had been getting into fights, most recently with her husband, presumably over money to buy drugs, and was verbalizing serious suicidal intentions. He had been hospitalized psychiatrically twice for depression and suicidal behavior during the past year after his girlfriend had left him. He acknowledged having a long history of cocaine and marijuana abuse, and had been on a crack binge just before the fight with his sister's husband. He also admitted to having once been arrested on an assault charge, but said that he was released from jail when the charge was dropped.

By the end of the first week of hospitalization, Mr. C.'s depression appeared to be steadily improving. However, he began to complain increasingly about nervousness, and to demand benzodiazepine, even though he was already receiving another anxiolytic medication and did not appear to manifest symptoms of anxiety. He became aggressive, demanding, and verbally abusive; exhibited intimidating behavior and engaged in frequent arguments with other patients; and constantly complained about the treatment he was receiving, particularly about the attitude of the staff in withholding medication from him. He insisted that he was not well enough to leave the ward, and threatened that if he were discharged, he would resume using drugs and would do terrible things, such as getting into fights and hurting people. One morning, after the nurse who was dispensing medication to the patients on the ward refused his demand for diazepine, he shouted obscenities at her and pushed her against the wall, bruising her shoulder, in an attempt to grab some of the medication. Security guards were summoned, and they assisted in getting the situation under control.

Later that day, an interdisciplinary disposition conference was convened by a senior staff psychiatrist in order to determine the best course of action in this case. A careful and systematic evaluation was conducted, which included interviewing Mr. C. and assessing his mental state, risk factors for violent behavior, and "differential dangerousness" on the ward and out of the hospital. After taking these factors into consideration, as well as a report from another staff nurse about his similar demands and behavior while a patient at another hospital, the senior psychiatrist and other conferees decided to discharge the patient, even though he insisted on staying in the hospital. Importantly, the patient was judged not to be psychotic, severely depressed, or suicidal, but to have long-standing characterological problems with substance abuse propensities. When confronted with the discharge decision, Mr. C. became quite angry and verbally abusive, and threatened to sue the doctors and the hospital. Faced with the realization that the discharge decision would not be revoked, however, he eventually calmed down and agreed to accept a referral to a substance abuse program in the community.

*Discussion of Case 3*

There are several psychiatric–legal issues relevant to dealing with this character-disordered and substance-abusing patient. The patient was initially admitted to the psychiatric unit because he was judged to be a serious danger to himself. As his depression improved, he began to become aggressive, demanding, disruptive, and eventually assaultive. In general, increased numbers of patients with chronic severe character pathology, often having borderline personality organizations, may negatively affect hospital inpatient units in three ways: decreased milieu specificity because of the need to devote considerable time and energy to measures of control; increased staff regression, with intensification of countertransference, dependency needs, and emotional exhaustion resulting from role diffusion; and diminished cost-effectiveness as a result of reduced therapeutic effectiveness and staff burnout (Johansen, 1983). From the patient's perspective, his further stay on the ward also could have a negative impact on him by promoting regressive tendencies in the form of more aggressive, demanding, and dangerous behaviors. Because of strong countertransference reactions that are often provoked among staff members in dealing with difficult patients, and violent ones in particular, and the need to ensure an unbiased and thorough evaluation of the case, a consultant who is not directly involved in the treatment of the patient may be of assistance in deciding whether or not to discharge a potentially violent individual.

In this regard, Schwartz and Pinsker (1987) describe the role of an independent examiner as someone able objectively to evaluate a patient's potential for dangerous behavior and to communicate his or her findings to the staff, thereby playing a mediating role in the resolution of the dispute between patient and staff. Travin and Bluestone (1987) describe an interdisciplinary disposition committee, composed of a senior consulting psychiatrist from outside the ward, preferably someone with forensic experience, and the psychiatric and other mental health professional staff members from the ward's therapeutic team, which conducts what is essentially a disposition hearing on the suitability of discharging a mentally compensated patient who is at high risk for violent behavior. A major indication for this hearing would be for a patient who had engaged in serious or repetitive dangerous behavior on the psychiatric ward. The chart is thoroughly reviewed, the patient is carefully interviewed, and the risk factors for dangerous behavior are systematically analyzed. Considerable time is spent on discussing the "differential dangerousness" of the patient on and off the ward. Although all members of the committee contribute details and varying perspectives on the case, it is the chief psychiatrist of the service who makes an initial decision, while the senior psychiatric consultant maintains the right of final decision. Having a senior psychiatrist provide consultation on whether or not to discharge patients who are identified as being at high risk for violence could be helpful in defending against a possible later charge of negligent release or third-party liability in the event of subsequent violent behavior by the patient on the outside.

In the above case, the interdisciplinary disposition committee concluded that Mr. C. had already received the maximum therapeutic benefits from his hospitalization, and that any further stay could, in fact, be detrimental to his condition. Importantly, the staff made an appointment for Mr. C. to attend a substance abuse program the next day, and learned, by telephone, that he kept his appointment. All of this was documented as evidence that could be used in forestalling or defending against a charge of abandonment of the patient.

## CONCLUSION

This chapter did not include an in-depth exploration of treatment approaches in the management of assaultive patients, but was meant to serve as a review of some of the major forensic considerations in this area. Implicit in this discussion has been the fundamental principle that good clinical practice necessarily respects the rights of both patients and staff members. Consequently, the emphasis has been on forensic aspects of managing assaultive patients, because clinical decision making about violent patients necessarily involves controlling these patients, and thus inherently risks violating the patient's rights in an attempt to control violent behavior. As this chapter has made clear, decision making in this area must encompass a keen attention to legal considerations, as well as to clinical concerns. Only by bringing both legal and clinical knowledge and concerns to bear on decision making in the management of violent patients can patients' need for treatment be met at the same time as their rights as individuals are maintained.

## REFERENCES

Adler, W. N., Kreeger, C., & Ziegler, P. (1983). Patient violence in a private psychiatric hospital. In J. R. Lion & W. H. Reid (Eds.), *Assaults within psychiatric facilities* (pp. 81–89). Orlando, FL: Grune & Stratton.

Appelbaum, P. S. (1983). Legal considerations in the prevention and treatment of assault. In J. R. Lion & W. H. Reid (Eds.), *Assaults within psychiatric facilities* (pp. 173–190). Orlando, FL: Grune & Stratton.

Appelbaum, P. S. (1987). Legal aspects of violence by psychiatric patients. In K. Tardiff (Section Ed.), *Annual review: Vol. 6. Violence and the violent patient* (pp. 549–564). Washington, DC: American Psychiatric Press.

Appelbaum, P. S., & Gutheil, T. G. (1991). *Clinical handbook of psychiatry and the law* (2d ed.). Baltimore, MD: Williams & Wilkins.

Appleton, W. S. (1965). The snow phenomenon: Tranquilizing the assaultive patient. *Psychiatry, 28,* 88–93.

Binder, R. L. (1979). The use of seclusion on an inpatient crisis intervention unit. *Hospital and Community Psychiatry, 30,* 266–269.

Binder, R. L., & McNeil, D. E. (1986). Victims and families of violent psychiatric patients. *Bulletin of the American Academy of Psychiatry and the Law, 14,* 131–139.

Brizer, D. A. (1989). Introduction: Overview of current approaches to the prediction of violence. In D. A. Brizer & M. Crowner (Eds.), *Current approaches to the prediction of violence* (pp. XI–XXIII). Washington, DC: American Psychiatric Press.

Craig, T. J. (1982). An epidemiologic study of problems associated with violence among psychiatric inpatients. *American Journal of Psychiatry, 139,* 1262–1266.

Davis, S. (1991). Violence by psychiatric inpatients: A review. *Hospital and Community Psychiatry, 42,* 585–590.

Dix, G. E. (1987). Legal and ethical issues in the treatment and handling of violent behavior. In L. H. Roth (Ed.), *Clinical treatment of the violent person* (pp. 178–206). New York: Guilford.

Dubin, W. R., & Stolberg, R. (1981). *Emergency psychiatry for the house officer.* New York: Spectrum.

Gutheil, T. G. (1985). Prosecuting patients. *Hospital and Community Psychiatry, 36,* 1320–1321.

Gutheil, T. G., & Tardiff, K. (1984). Indications and contraindications for seclusion and restraint. In K. Tardiff (Ed.), *The psychiatric uses of seclusion and restraint* (pp. 11–17). Washington, DC: American Psychiatric Press.

Halleck, S. L. (1980). *Law in the practice of psychiatry: A handbook for clinicians.* New York: Plenum.

Haller, R. M., & Deluty, R. H. (1988). Assaults on staff by psychiatric inpatients: A critical review. *British Journal of Psychiatry, 152,* 174–179.

Hanke, N. (1984). *Handbook of emergency psychiatry.* Lexington, MA: Heath.

Johansen, K. H. (1983). The impact of patients with chronic character pathology on a hospital inpatient unit. *Hospital and Community Psychiatry, 34,* 842–846.

Lee, H. K., Villar, O., Juthani, N., & Bluestone, H. (1989). Characteristics and behavior of patients involved in psychiatric ward incidents. *Hospital and Community Psychiatry, 40,* 1295–1297.

Lion, J. R., & Soloff, P. H. (1984). Implementation of seclusion and restraint. In K. Tardiff (Ed.), *The psychiatric uses of seclusion and restraint* (pp. 19–34). Washington, DC: American Psychiatric Press.

McNeil, D. E., & Binder, R. L. (1987). Predictive validity of judgments of dangerousness in emergency civil commitment. *American Journal of Psychiatry, 144,* 197–200.

Miller, R. D., & Maier, G. J. (1987). Factors affecting the decision to prosecute mental patients for criminal behavior. *Hospital and Community Psychiatry, 38,* 50–55.

New York Mental Hygiene Law, sec. 33.04 (McKinney, 1988 & Supp. 1992).

*New York Official Compilation of Codes, Rules, and Regulations,* tit. 14, sec. 27.7 (1986).

Phelan, L. A., Mills, M. J., & Ryan, J. A. (1985). Prosecuting psychiatric patients for assault. *Hospital and Community Psychiatry, 36,* 581–582.

Plutchik, R., Karasu, T. B., Conte, H. R., Siegel, B., & Jerrett, I. (1978). Toward a rationale for the seclusion process. *Journal of Nervous and Mental Disease, 166,* 571–579.

Reid, W. H., Bolinger, M. F., & Edwards, J. G. (1989). Serious assaults by inpatients. *Psychosomatics, 30,* 54–56.

Rofman, E. S., Askinazi, C., & Fant, E. (1980). The prediction of dangerous behavior in emergency civil commitment. *American Journal of Psychiatry, 137,* 1061–1064.

*Rogers v. Okin,* 478 F.Supp. 1342 (1979).

Rossi, A. M., Jacobs, M., Monteleone, M., Olsen, R., Surber, R. W., Winkler, E. L., & Wommack, A. (1985). Violent or fear-inducing behavior associated with hospital admission. *Hospital and Community Psychiatry, 36,* 643–647.

Schwartz, H. I., & Pinsker, H. (1987). Mediating retention or release of the potentially dangerous patient. *Hospital and Community Psychiatry, 38,* 75–77.

Simon, R. I. (1987). *Clinical psychiatry and the law.* Washington, DC: American Psychiatric Press.

Soloff, P. H. (1987). Physical controls: The use of seclusion and restraint in modern psychiatric practice. In L. H. Roth (Ed.), *Clinical treatment of the violent person* (pp. 119–137). New York: Guilford.

Soloff, P. H., Gutheil, T. G., & Wexler, D. B. (1985). Seclusion and restraint in 1985: A review and update. *Hospital and Community Psychiatry, 36,* 652–657.

Tardiff, K. (1981). Emergency control measures for psychiatric inpatients. *Journal of Nervous and Mental Disease, 169,* 614–618.

Tardiff, K. (Ed.). (1984). *The psychiatric uses of seclusion and restraint.* Washington, DC: American Psychiatric Press.

Tardiff, K. (1991). Violence by psychiatric patients. In R. I. Simon (Ed.), *Review of clinical psychiatry and the law* (Vol. 2) (pp. 175–233). Washington, DC: American Psychiatric Press.

Travin, S., & Bluestone, H. (1987). Discharging the violent psychiatric inpatient. *Journal of Forensic Sciences, 32,* 999–1008.

Tupin, J. P. (1983). The violent patient: A strategy for management and diagnosis. *Hospital and Community Psychiatry, 34,* 37–40.

Wadeson, H., & Carpenter, W. T. (1976). Impact of the seclusion room experience. *Journal of Nervous and Mental Disease, 163,* 318–328.

Wexler, D. B. (1984). Legal aspects of seclusion and restraint. In K. Tardiff (Ed.), *The psychiatric uses of seclusion and restraint* (pp. 111–124). Washington, DC: American Psychiatric Press.

Yesavage, J. A., & Brizer, D. A. (1989). Clinical and historical correlates of dangerous inpatient behavior. In D. A. Brizer & M. Crowner (Eds.), *Current approaches to the prediction of violence* (pp. 65–84). Washington, DC: American Psychiatric Press.

*Youngberg v. Romeo,* 102 S.Ct. 2452 (1982).

# 6

# Inpatient Geriatric Psychiatry
## Special Legal and
## Ethical Considerations

KAREN BLANK AND
HAROLD I. SCHWARTZ

Over the past two decades, the population of persons 65 years old and older has grown at a rate twice as fast as the general population. The group aged 85 and older is the fastest growing portion of the population, increasing 165 percent from 1960 to 1982. Future projections indicate that while the total U.S. population is expected to grow by 33 percent between 1982 and 2050, the over-55 group is projected to grow by 113 percent (Stein, 1988). The enormous growth in the elderly population has been accompanied by a persistently negative attitude toward the aged that leaves this group subject to mistreatment and discrimination. This unfortunate situation is compounded for the mentally ill elderly, who are essentially doubly demeaned in our culture. Not surprisingly, the presence of the mentally ill elderly is increasing on inpatient psychiatric units. As many as 25 percent of all treatment episodes of psychiatrically ill elderly occur in the inpatient services of general hospitals (Barton & Barton, 1983), and specialized inpatient geropsychiatry units have been developed in some centers to address the needs of this population.

Many of the legal and ethical issues raised within the course of general psychiatric care seem to be even more compelling in the treatment of the elderly. There are a multitude of forces, from attitudinal to institutional, that have the effect of compromising the autonomy and self-determination of elderly persons during the course of treatment for psychiatric disorders and dementing illnesses. The psychiatric practitioner must be cognizant of the legal and ethical issues involved in geriatric psychiatric care so as best to be able to provide quality care for patients, while respecting their rights.

## INFORMED CONSENT AND TREATMENT DECISIONS

The concept of informed consent is critical to the understanding of almost all of the special forensic considerations pertaining to the psychiatric hospitalization of geriatric patients. It is an issue at the point of consent to hospitalization, at each significant treatment decision, and around discharge planning. The informed-consent doctrine has transformed the doctor–patient relationship in recent decades, shifting the balance of power in treatment decisions to the patient (Schwartz & Roth, 1989). This shift has occurred within the lifetimes of older patients, whose earlier experiences with the medical profession took place in the age of beneficent paternalism. Physicians commonly made treatment decisions without including the patient. By definition, the paternalistic physician behaved much like a parent, deciding for the infantilized and dependent child. Some elderly patients retain the expectation that physicians and patients should behave in this manner. Haug (1979) found that patients over the age of 60 are more likely to accept physician authority without challenge.

Certain elements in the doctor–older patient relationship may work to the detriment of informed consent in treatment decisions. The patient's expectations of this relationship may lead him or her too readily to waive informed-consent efforts altogether. Such waivers should be explored, and usually discouraged. Also to be considered are the myriad transference and countertransference reactions that can arise in the elderly patient–physician dyad, all of which can discourage adherence to the informed-consent doctrine. For example, there are fragile, depressed, helpless patients who evoke in the physician feelings of omnipotent control. Other elderly patients may attempt to infantilize the physician, causing the physician to become either overly controlling or less competent and physicianly. The help-rejecting patient or hostile delusional patient can demand enormous expenditures of physician energy, which can lead the clinician to feel irritated, less empathic, and less disposed to respect the patient's wishes. Obviously, the clinician must monitor such reactions to minimize their effects on adherence to the informed-consent doctrine. Conscious or unconscious ageism on the clinician's part may also erode the process.

At the core of the informed-consent doctrine is recognition of the individual's fundamental right to self-determination and personal autonomy (Kapp & Bigot, 1985; President's Commission, 1982). The competent patient's decisions must be respected; the patient retains control over his or her own body, protected from unwanted intrusions. It can be argued that self-determination should be, if anything, more respected as a patient ages (Gaylin, 1982). Older patients have a wealth of life experiences and established values upon which they can draw when needed to render important health decisions.

Competency is the cornerstone of informed consent. Two points must be kept in mind when evaluating a patient's competency. First, the psychiatrist provides a determination about *clinical* competency (de facto competency or decisional capacity). This clinical finding may inform a proceeding to determine a patient's legal (de jure) competency, but physicians do not, themselves, determine legal competency. Second, the evaluation of competency must be made regarding competency for specific tasks or decisions (Ciccone & Clements, 1987). Use of the term "decisional capacity" emphasizes the decision-specific nature of clinical competency. Global competency is seldom a useful concept in the clinical context.

While the legal criteria for decisional capacity to consent to treatment are not uniformly defined (Appelbaum & Gutheil, 1982), the consensus of case law and ethical principle generally requires that the patient have an understanding of his or her medical situation and the proposed treatment's risks, benefits, and alternatives. In practice, the requirement that a patient demonstrate factual understanding is often experienced as an overly stringent and impractical standard for certain decisions, especially for treatments that carry little risk and great benefit. A number of studies suggest that significant numbers of patients who consent to treatment do not understand them factually (Grossman & Summers, 1980; Olin & Olin, 1975). In practice, the distinction between a patient's ability to understand and actual understanding (as demonstrated by the patient) is often blurred. Of course, the greater the risk the treatment involves, the more exacting and stringent the physician should be in obtaining fully informed consent (Schwartz & Roth, 1989).

There is controversy as to the effects of aging in general on the ability to give informed consent. However, it is hazardous to generalize the abilities of the aged as they are a markedly heterogeneous group. Having said this, we must note the finding by Taub (1980) of some impairment in the ability of "normal" older individuals to remember consent information. In comparing the aged with younger medical patients, Stanley, Stanley, and Pomara (1985) found generally poorer understanding of consent information for research participation and less reasonable decision making (as manifested by agreeing to participate more often in a high-risk/low-benefit study). This tendency was further increased in the cognitively impaired.

It is important to consider clinical competency to be a fluid rather than static capacity. Decisional capacity is not always clearly present or absent, but it may fluctuate according to the complexity of the decision being faced, the manner of communication of this decision, and the state of the patient's illness (Ciccone & Clements, 1987; Schwartz & Blank, 1986).

A 60-year-old retired, single seamstress with a history of depression responsive to electroconvulsive therapy (ECT) 15 years earlier was hospitalized for a severe depression characterized by somatic delusions, delusions of poverty, and a suicide attempt. Despite her psychosis, she was able to give fully informed consent for ECT after careful explanation. After 12 treatments, she was no longer depressed or delusional, but remained mistrustful and isolated. This apparently was consistent with her baseline personality. She showed mild cognitive impairment, especially of short-term memory, consistent with a post-ECT effect. Days before her discharge, she suddenly began to complain of back pain and intermittent urinary incontinence. Examination revealed abnormal lower-extremity reflexes and x-rays showed worsening compression of a preexisting T12 vertebral collapse.

An immediate myelogram was recommended. Under this stress, the patient became increasingly paranoid, stating that she did not believe that anything was wrong with her back and that the staff was urging her to have the myelogram in order to torture her, out of revenge for having been a difficult patient. Although she had been felt to be clinically competent despite her psychosis when deciding about ECT, at this point her reasoning was impaired by delusional beliefs. She showed no evidence of understanding her condition, the recommended procedure, or the risks of refusing it. It was only after a medical student who was trusted by the patient spent more than an hour with her, explaining her condition and the staff's concerns and drawing schematic diagrams of her spinal cord and the procedure, that the patient was able to demonstrate understanding of the risks and benefits and to make an informed decision.

Older persons, when stressed, may fearfully avoid new situations that threaten to overwhelm their precarious coping strategies. They may initially refuse critical, lifesaving treatment, and give the appearance of making an illogical and incompetent decision. It is crucial for the physician to assist in developing an environment in which the patient will be optimally receptive to information (Sadoff, 1991; Schwartz & Blank, 1986). Shifts in competency are quite common. For example, when decisional incapacity is attributable to the psychiatric illness under treatment, that treatment may restore the patient to full clinical competency. Alternatively, patients who start out clinically competent may temporarily need substitute decision makers, as in the example of patients being rendered temporarily incapacitated by memory impairment from ECT. Decisional capacity needs to be reassessed frequently depending on the patient's clinical condition and the decision at hand. In complicated situations, consultation with legal counsel may be invaluable in forming decisions that are both clinically and legally sound.

Although the literature on competency evaluations is voluminous, such evaluations cannot be strictly standardized; by their very nature, they are inextricably linked to the situation at hand. The emphasis should not be placed merely on the objective nature of the specific decision made and whether or not it agrees with the physician's recommendations, but rather on the capacity of the patient and the quality of the thought processes followed in arriving at the decision (Meisel, Roth, & Lidz, 1977). It is essential that the psychiatrist carefully document the content of the patient's decisional capacity evaluation, avoiding global or solely conclusory statements.

## Substitute Decision Making

When elderly psychiatric inpatients are not able to make informed choices, they may be considered to be clinically incompetent (to lack decisional capacity). Substituted consent must be obtained, either from a family member, through formal guardianship proceedings, by court order, or by other mechanisms required by statute or regulation. Many statutes that govern informed consent and involvement of family are quite unclear and leave much open to interpretation. At one extreme, some jurisdictions require formal judicial proceedings for most significant treatment decisions involving the decisionally incapacitated patient. To treat without such a hearing might constitute grounds for battery. Other areas grant much more latitude in using family judgments to proceed with treatment.

Guardians may be appointed by the courts to make decisions on behalf of a legally incompetent person regarding his or her person or estate. A number of different guardianship arrangements exist. A plenary guardian has authority for making decisions in virtually every area of the ward's life—finances, where the ward will reside, and medical issues, for example. Alternatively, guardianship powers can be restricted to specific areas, such as control of financial assets or health-care decisions. Such arrangements are often referred to as conservatorships. Alternatively, the courts can assign a guardian ad litem who has authority to represent the incompetent person only in a particular legal proceeding. Fortunately, the courts are moving away from considering competency a global, all-or-nothing phenomenon, and, in many jurisdictions, provide the possibility of partial guardianships or conservatorships, in which the court delineates the specific areas over which the guardian retains discretion (Kapp & Bigot, 1985). Obviously, a health-care professional must become aware of the extent and limits of the guardian's or conservator's powers before entrusting him or her with medical decisions (Kapp & Bigot, 1985).

## ADMISSION TO THE HOSPITAL

The decision as to whether to admit an elderly patient to a psychiatric unit should be a carefully considered one. Abruptly removing a patient from his or her familiar surroundings may have serious deleterious effects. Efforts to avoid hospitalization should be made by assessing and treating the patient in the community whenever possible (Bluestone, Travin, & Kaufman, 1987). Elderly patients who are admitted to psychiatric facilities often share some characteristics that set them apart from their younger cohorts. For the majority, it is their first experience with psychiatric admission. Elderly patients more often live alone or in institutions (Ross & Kedward, 1977). In addition, they more often have physical limitations, medical problems, and sensory deficits. The unit milieu should have the capacity to adapt to these special needs.

When a patient voluntarily admits himself or herself to a psychiatric facility, his or her competency to make this decision is usually not challenged. When a patient cooperates with voluntary admission, in accordance with a physician's recommendations, he or she is viewed as behaving in such a way as to promote a reasonable outcome. Since the patient is entitled to care under the least restrictive setting and commitment proceedings can be cumbersome, the patient's assent is often accepted, and the ability to make this decision is usually not questioned. In clinical practice, an impaired patient is voluntarily hospitalized if the patient so assents by his or her behavior and there is no conflict among the patient, caregiver, and family (Baker & Finkel, 1988). The American Psychiatric Association (1983) has published guidelines that condone the voluntary admission of assenting patients who apparently lack decisional capacity if the consent of a guardian or next of kin is acquired. The guidelines require the clinician to attempt to obtain informed consent from the patient as his or her condition improves. However, there are studies that suggest that a significant number of people presenting themselves for voluntary admission to a public mental hospital are seriously compromised, rendering the giving of truly informed consent unlikely, if not impossible (Appelbaum, Mirkin, & Bateman, 1981). In *Zinermon v. Burch* (1990), the U.S. Supreme Court rejected the practice of accepting the assent of possibly incompetent patients, endorsing efforts to ascertain the competency of patients prior to obtaining consent for hospitalization. Given that many states already require that patients consenting to hospitalization be competent to do so, and the subtle and complex nature of competency assessments, it is unclear as to what actual impact this decision will have on clinical practice.

Questions of competency are most often raised when the patient and the clinician disagree about the need for hospitalization. Seriously ill elderly patients, especially those suffering from depressive disorders, resist hospitalization for a number of reasons (Blank, 1987). An understanding of these reasons can allow the admitting psychiatrist to explore the meaning of hospitalization with the patient, and sometimes to avoid commitment. Obviously, considerable prejudice against and fear of psychiatric treatment exist, and can be exacerbated in some older patients as compared with their younger peers. Past associations of psychiatric facilities with long-term sanitoriums, state hospitals, or "snake pits" can be resurrected. Whether their trepidations are based in reality or fantasy, some patients may fear that the implications of being diagnosed as "insane" may be used against them in future guardianship or conservatorship proceedings. Patients may also associate hospitalization with serious illness and death, or view it as the avenue through which they will be coerced into a nursing home. In addition, refusal of hospitalization, in general, can result from some elderly persons' adoption of a position of increased conservatism and inflexibility. When this occurs, the person fearfully avoids new surroundings as they may overwhelm coping abilities and present him or her with new, unmanageable emotional and financial stressors. These types of understandable fears are exacerbated by the commonly occurring geriatric disorders of depression and dementia.

When questions do exist about the patient's competency, the physician should evaluate the patient's decisional capacity, not globally, but specifically regarding the decision to sign into the hospital. When a patient is not competent to make this decision, civil commitment or short-term emergency hospitalization should be arranged. Since the legal requirements and procedures for involuntary admission differ according to jurisdiction, physicians must be familiar with the applicable regulations.

## Commitment

Commitment to a psychiatric facility occurs for a significant minority of elderly patients. In one setting, 22% of psychiatric inpatients over the age of 65 were admitted involuntarily (Blank, Vingiano, & Schwartz, 1989). As in the case of younger patients, involuntary hospitalization is governed by one of two principles, depending on the jurisdiction and clinical presentation: police powers (commitment criteria based on dangerousness) and *parens patriae* powers ("father of the land" criteria based on the state's benevolently treating those who cannot or will not protect themselves) (Kapp & Bigot, 1985). Concerns have been raised about the appropriateness of both criteria with regard to elderly patients. The use of broader *parens patriae* powers to commit elderly patients has raised concerns that they may be committed inappropriately. Jones, Parlour, and Badger (1982) found this to be the case with patients committed to state facilities. Tomelleri, Lakshminawayanan, and Herjanic (1977) discovered that a higher proportion of patients aged 70 years and over were involuntarily hospitalized through court commitments as compared with younger patients. However, this higher rate of commitment in the older patient population was not found in studies by Munetz, Kaufman, and Rich (1980); Okin (1986); and Zwerdling, Karasu, Plutchik, and Kellerman (1975). Inappropriate commitment of the elderly, where it does exist, is becoming a special concern considering the increasing numbers of organically impaired elderly individuals and the relative paucity of appropriate nursing-home facilities and home-care resources to support this population.

While some states have adopted commitment criteria based on the inability to care for oneself rather than dangerousness (Miller, 1990a), the majority of commitment statutes enacted during the past decades have generally required a showing of dangerousness as a prerequisite for involuntary hospitalization (Brakel, Parry, & Weiner, 1985; Roth, 1980; Schwitzgebel & Schwitzgebel, 1980). These more stringent and narrowly defined commitment criteria are more difficult to apply toward securing treatment for the elderly than are the broader *parens patriae* criteria. The conditions that often afflict older persons, such as dementia, psychotic disorders, and serious mood disturbances, can result in marked impairments in self-care without convincingly causing dangerous behaviors when these are strictly defined. In those states with more stringent legal requirements for commitment, obtaining hospitalization for patients unable to care for themselves can be difficult, particularly for patients who lack family or other involved advocates to petition the court. Indeed, the *Zinermon v. Burch* decision could create a class of patients who, lacking competency to consent to hospitalization but failing to meet dangerousness criteria for commitment, are not hospitalizable (Miller, 1990b).

In a study done in a state with a broad *parens patriae* commitment statute, it was found that physicians appropriately committed elderly patients, conforming to the regulations, without the need for formal judicial intervention. All of the patients were gravely ill and in need of psychiatric hospitalization, but some of them probably would not have been hospitalized under commitment statutes requiring a showing of overt dangerousness.

Mrs. Z. was an 82-year-old former nightclub singer who was diagnosed as having senile dementia of the Alzheimers type and was cared for at home by her husband, who also was undergoing a cognitive decline, though to a lesser extent. She had insulin-dependent diabetes as well, and suffered from atrial fibrillation, which was managed with digoxin. Mrs. Z. had a history of several months of intermittent delusional beliefs that her husband was an imposter and a kidnapper, but her husband was generally able to reassure her or distract her when she became frightened by these ideas. During the week prior to her admission, she became difficult to manage at home. She often failed to recognize her husband or became terrified that he was an imposter, and she would run out on her lawn, screaming for help. While she usually allowed him to administer insulin, she became increasingly combative around this issue and her food intake became erratic. She demanded that she be permitted to administer her own cardiac medication, to which he reluctantly agreed, unsure that she could do it properly. Her behavior became increasingly agitated, especially at night. She refused to take the "new medicine," haloperidol, that her internist prescribed by phone. The geriatric psychiatrist contacted by the internist was concerned about the possibility of delirium, as well as worsening of Mrs. Z.'s dementia, and recommended involuntary hospitalization.

This case illustrates the inadequacy of strict "dangerousness" criteria when considering the need for hospitalization for many geriatric patients. While this patient was clearly gravely disabled, and likely to deteriorate seriously in the near future, she would not meet criteria for dangerousness in those jurisdictions that require overt findings of suicidality or homicidality. In order for commitment laws to provide optimal applicability for the aged, their criteria need to include such provisions as "inability to care for self" and "grave disability" (Blank et al., 1989).

Finally, a potential clinical hazard with significant medicolegal consequences involves the failure of the clinician to admit an elderly patient because of a tendency to underestimate the patient's actual suicide potential. The same hazard exists with regard to evaluations of the appropriateness of discharge. Suicide rates are higher among persons over age 65 than among their younger cohorts. In 1984, the suicide rate for the general population was 11.6 per 100,000 and the rate for white men age 65 and older was 41.6, nearly four times the national rate (Warheit, Longino, & Bradsher, 1991). Countertransference and ageistic attitudes may interfere with the accurate assessment of suicidality. An elderly, frail patient may harbor suicidal ideas that are underappreciated or overlooked by the physician if the physician's bias is that elderly persons tend not to take such drastic, decisive measures. Alternatively, the physician could overlook the role of a depressive illness and could unconsciously, or even consciously, collude with the patient's professed belief that he or she has lived long enough and that his or her suffering should end.

## CONFIDENTIALITY

The ethical duty of maintaining confidentiality has always been essential to patient care. While there are legitimate exceptions to the principle of confidentiality, most commonly lapses are secondary to careless clinical practice. Maintaining the confidentiality of an elderly hospitalized patient is a complex issue; numerous members of the treatment team need information about the patient, and the patient's family is often highly involved. Psychiatrists must be careful to disclose only that which is necessary for inpatient staff to function effectively with the patient (Simon, 1987). While family involvement is often critical to successful treatment, it is recommended that therapists obtain express, written permission from the patient whenever possible before sharing information with the family (Eth, 1991). In inpatient clinical practice, this is seldom done, and often assumptions are made for the patient about the degree to which the family should be involved. Elderly patients are not infrequently deprived of privacy and of confidential relationships with their therapists as a result. Such ethical violations can have unfortunate clinical consequences. For example, when the patient is paranoid, unexpected violations of confidentiality can spell doom for the therapeutic alliance. Clinicians must take great care to inform the patient about the nature of the doctor–patient relationship and the limits of confidentiality. In addition, it is the responsibility of physicians to be aware of statutes or regulations in their areas that mandate the reporting of information about elder abuse to protective services or of Alzheimer's disease to the motor vehicle bureau (Eth, 1991).

## SPECIAL LEGAL CONSIDERATIONS IN TREATMENT

### Diagnosis

The presentations of psychiatric disorders in the elderly often differ significantly from those in younger patients, introducing very real liability risk for failure to make the correct diagnosis. In the diagnosis of depression, for example, common errors include failing to recognize the etiologic role of physical illness or medication side effects, failing to diagnose "masked depression" in a patient presenting with physical complaints, failing to recognize depression in the physically ill, and failing to diagnose depression when dementia is the predominant symptomatic picture.

A myriad of diagnostic pitfalls also confronts the psychiatrist working with the organically impaired patient, the most serious among them being the failure to recognize delirium as a psychiatric emergency and the overlooking of treatable causes of dementia that can occur in approximately 15–20 percent of demented patients. Consultation with a geriatric psychiatrist should be obtained when diagnostic uncertainty exists.

**Psychotropic Medication**

Somatic treatments bring with them special and often serious risks that can only be highlighted in the context of this chapter. It is essential that the treating physician be well trained in geriatric psychopharmacology if he or she treats older persons. If this is not the case, consultation with a geriatric psychiatrist is indicated. Cyclic antidepressants are frequently used in this age group, and they require modifications of selection, dosage, dosing schedule, and monitoring. The risks of these medications for the elderly differ from and are usually more severe than those for younger patients. For example, sedation when combined with hypotension can contribute to falls and fractures. Hypotension alone can lead to falls, strokes, and myocardial infarction. Sinus tachycardia can jeopardize a patient with significant limitations of cardiac reserve, and the quinidine-like effect of these medications can produce a variety of serious conduction defects. Anticholinergic toxicity can pose serious problems for the elderly, such as urinary retention, precipitation of narrow-angle glaucoma, and full-blown central anticholinergic delirium (Salzman, 1984). Lithium, monoamine oxidase inhibitors, and the newer generation of antidepressants all have important roles in the treatment of geriatric patients, but similarly carry with them special risks for this age group (Salzman, 1984).

Neuroleptic medication is frequently used, and unfortunately sometimes overused, with geriatric patients. The risks are numerous and will not be covered here in detail. Tardive dyskinesia (TD), however, deserves special mention. Advanced age is the most powerful predictor for the development of TD (Saltz et al., 1989). Saltz has found the incidence of TD to be up to 40 percent after 40 weeks of cumulative neuroleptic exposure in patients over 55 (Saltz et al., 1989). Jeste and Wyatt (1982) report that the overall weighted mean prevalence of TD for patients over the age of 40 is nearly three times that of those under 40 years of age. Moreover, research suggests that TD becomes more severe and more persistent with aging (Smith & Baldessarini, 1980). Because the risks of neuroleptic exposure are great, the use of these agents requires particularly careful adherence to the informed-consent doctrine.

## Electroconvulsive Therapy

It is well documented that in the depressed geriatric population ECT is often the treatment of choice (Kramer, 1987; Weiner, 1982). Despite overwhelming evidence of its safety and efficacy, the regulatory atmosphere regarding this treatment has become increasingly severe (Winslade, 1988). At least half of the states have specific statutes or regulations that are generally designed to ensure the patient's informed consent and to protect the right to refuse this treatment. Many states lump ECT with psychosurgery, requiring a court order, appointment of a conservator, or some other legal procedure before treatment may be administered to an incompetent patient. It is vital that the physician be familiar with the regulations in his or her jurisdiction regarding the administration of ECT to the decisionally incapacitated patient.

A 76-year-old widow with a well-documented history of recurrent major depression was transferred to an inpatient unit from her residential treatment facility for treatment of a depressive illness. During this four-month-long episode, she had taken to bed, refusing almost all nutrition, bathing, and participation in social activities. In the days preceding admission, she expressed the delusional belief that her intestines were gangrenous and that she was destitute (even though she was secure financially). A psychiatrist at her residential facility had initially prescribed haloperididol and nortriptylene, but dosages were limited because of extrapyramidal and hypotensive effects. She had responded favorably to ECT for a similar, though less severe, episode six years earlier. When the inpatient staff recommended ECT, she refused it, claiming that it would be of no use because of the condition of her intestines, and that she could not afford the treatments and needed to be transferred immediately to the "poor house." While the staff attempted another pharmacologic course, the patient's condition worsened; she began refusing virtually all food and most fluids, and expressed the wish to die. Her children agreed to ECT after being fully informed, and the staff commenced ECT treatment after following the applicable state regulatory requirements (having an outside consultant and the chief of service examine the patient's clinical competency and agree as to the need for ECT). After her third ECT, showing no detectable memory impairment, she gave informed consent for continuing the treatments. She responded fully to eight unilateral treatments and returned to her residential facility.

In all cases, the clinician should carefully document the process of obtaining informed consent for ECT. The memory impairment that may occur as an ECT side effect highlights the fact that informed consent is an ongoing process. Efforts must be made to maintain the patient's knowledge of the procedure and consent throughout the treatment. Involvement of family members in this process may be critical.

**Restraints**

The use of physical restraints raises special problems in the aged patient. While restraints are more often encountered in nursing homes or medical hospital settings, from 7% to 85%, depending on the setting (Strumpf & Evans, 1988; Tinetti, Liu, Marottoli, & Ginter, 1991), they are also used in inpatient psychiatric settings. In distinction to their use in younger psychiatric patients, restraints for the elderly are used less often for violent behavior and more often for the prevention of falls. It is important to recognize that the effectiveness of restraints in the prevention of falls and injuries is not at all clear. Restraints do, however, carry very real risks of their own. They are a major offense to the dignity and autonomy of older persons, and subject them to morbidity from immobilization and accidental injury from the restraint itself.

Mrs. S., an 83-year-old retired businesswoman, had known great success in her career and had worked in the family exporting business she had founded until her Alzheimer's disease became incapacitating. She required hospitalization after her dementia became complicated by paranoid delusions accompanied by violent outbursts consisting primarily of trying to strike people with her cane. Screaming at passersby in German, her native language, she would attempt to strike out, sometimes losing her balance and toppling backwards. Her physician would frequently request x-ray studies after these falls, often needing to sedate her heavily for the procedures. A variety of pharmacologic interventions were attempted, including neuroleptics and buspirone, but had side effects and were of only limited value in modifying her outbursts. The staff finally decided on a schedule of restraint in a cardiac chair in order to maintain the milieu and the patient's safety. Unfortunately, the length of time of each restraint episode steadily increased until the patient was spending the most of each day in restraints. This once regal appearing woman rapidly lost much of her remaining language skills (too rapidly to be accounted for by the normal progression of her disease), constantly moaned and cried out, and became incontinent. She had, up until the restraints, been able to use the bathroom with assistance. Fortunately, her family was able to secure a place for her in an excellent nursing facility that rarely used restraints. The staff there elected to forgo restraints and risk possible injury, viewing it as an unfortunate complication of her decline. Within the nursing home milieu, she fared reasonably well.

Whereas very short-term use to prevent injury may be unavoidable at times, it is important for the clinician to determine the true motivation for the restraint, including a careful consideration of the role of fear of litigation. Of note, no lawsuit has been successful against an institution simply for failure to restrain (Strumpf & Evans, 1988). Wherever possible, the patient and family should be included in the decision as to whether to use physical restraints or to accept the risks of not restraining.

## DISCHARGE PLANNING

Discharge planning presents some of the thorniest clinical, legal, and ethical problems in caring for elderly psychiatric inpatients. Recommendations for placement or for the use of home health aides have a profound impact on the patient's liberty, autonomous functioning, and privacy. Unlike the treatment-planning process, where the patient's current capacities and judgments are the focus, projections of future abilities are crucial to discharge-planning decisions (Dubler, 1988). Dubler has succinctly stated the problem in this regard: "Assessment of future risk to patient, family and community requires prognostic skills only granted to soothsayers and purveyors of crystal balls." As hospital stays shorten, the patient's projected recovery condition is often quite discrepant with his or her condition and abilities at the time of discharge. Furthermore, the hospital is a particularly hazardous setting in which to measure future abilities (Dubler, 1988); the side effects of hospitalization, such as excessive dependency in the service of the sick role, sleep disruptions, fear, and loneliness, all may act further to compromise the patient's condition, decisional abilities, and choices.

Another necessary but complicating issue is the role of the family in discharge planning. When patients render informed decisions about their medical treatment, it is their right to refuse input from family members. In contrast, discharge-planning decisions often significantly affect the rights and responsibilities of family members. Families cannot be enlisted into a discharge plan as care givers without their willingness to participate, nor can families coerce patients into a plan for their own convenience.

Mrs. T., an 80-year-old woman, had been admitted at the urging of her son and her internist, who were alarmed at her worsening depression after she "took to bed" at the hotel where she was living. She stopped dressing and lost interest in all her previous pleasures. Her hospital workup documented moderate cognitive decline consistent with the senile dementia of the Alzheimer's type diagnosed before her move from Chicago four months earlier. However, most impressive was her rapid mood and behavioral improvement in the hospital without any pharmacologic intervention. She dressed herself on her second day, and began to take advantage of therapeutic activities with considerable relish. It rapidly became apparent that there was a family struggle, with the patient wanting to live in an adult facility or nursing home and her son, a distinguished attorney, opposing this idea. He was greatly horrified by the idea of a nursing home and at being "the type of person who would institutionalize his mother." Instead, he had transported her from her home in Chicago to a suite in one of New York's finest hotels and hired 24-hour nurses to tend her. The patient was isolated and bored in the hotel. The staff concluded that her decision to move to a health-related facility was a competent one, and advised the son that his mother's wishes were primary and should be respected. The disagreement between mother and son could not be worked out in the few days of hospitalization, and they were referred to a geriatric social worker to continue the process. The son continued to be determined to "try everything" to avoid placement, and the mother opted to stay at the hotel and not displease her son. Unfortunately, they attended only two sessions with the therapist and eventually were lost to follow-up.

A discharge plan must attempt to combine the patient's choices and best interests with what family, community, and funding sources will allow (Dubler, 1988). All patients who are competent, as well as those who, though somewhat compromised, are able to participate, must be informed about the available discharge options and must be given sufficient time and support to consider and decide among these options. At the culmination of this process, the decision of a competent patient must be respected, even if it involves the patient's assumption of some degree of personal risk.

In addition, it is the responsibility of the clinician to educate patients and their families about support in the community and about reimbursement procedures and entitlements. Utilization of such programs or funding sources can make a critical difference in ensuring continuation of recovery postdischarge, prevention of relapse, and avoidance of unnecessary placement.

Finally, it is extremely important that physicians, in collaboration with the social service staff, begin the process of legal and financial planning with patients who are suffering from dementia and the families of these patients. Early, sensitive discussion is of enormous benefit because it allows the patient to be maximally involved in making his or her own choices about the future. The patient may wish to make some financial and estate planning decisions, have input into his or her future health care and residence, or become a research participant.

The physician should possess a working knowledge of legal mechanisms, such as durable powers of attorney, living wills, and federal entitlement program requirements, and should provide the patient and family with referral to an attorney knowledgeable in these matters. Encouraging patients to play an active role in such planning obviously not only benefits the patient, but can be of ongoing help to the family member who must assume growing responsibility for making judgments on behalf of an increasingly demented relative.

## ELDER ABUSE

Whereas child abuse has deservedly been the focus of public and professional interest for some time, elder abuse has only recently begun to be recognized as a serious and common problem in our society. Inpatient and emergency room psychiatrists are well positioned to detect, intervene, and prevent continuation of elder abuse. Unfortunately, the expertise to do so is often lacking and opportunities for intervention can be lost.

Elderly persons are particularly vulnerable to abuse for many reasons. Abuse that occurs in the home is outside of scrutiny, and the more infirm or house-bound abused elderly are less likely to come to the attention of others. Studies indicate that lack of adequate resources is a major risk factor for abuse (Goldstein, 1989). The majority of elderly abuse victims have been found to be women over 75 who do not have sufficient financial resources to live independently (Goldstein, 1989) and have physical or mental impairments that interfere with their self-care. Kosberg (1987) describes six types of abuse in his comprehensive definition of elder abuse: (1) passive neglect; (2) active neglect; (3) verbal, emotional, or psychological abuse; (4) physical abuse; (5) material or financial misappropriation; and (6) violation of rights. Neglect of a passive nature has been shown to be the most common form of abuse (Goldstein, 1989). In 1981, a National Conference on Abuse of Older Persons concluded that 4% of the nation's elderly may be victims of some sort of moderate to severe abuse, though it is estimated that only one sixth of the cases come to the attention of authorities; that the abuse was likely to be recurrent; and that generally the abused older person lives with the abuser, who is a relative (Gardner &

Halamandaris, 1981). As older persons tend not to report their own abuse, it is imperative for mental health professionals to be sensitive to signs of abuse, to be trained in sensitively eliciting confirmatory information, and to know how to intervene.

> Shortly after the transfer of Mr. W. from the medical service to psychiatry, it became apparent to the staff that the dehydration and 35-pound weight loss that precipitated his admission was not due to depression but to possible neglect by his adult son. On the unit, Mr. W., a retired baker, was sociable and ate with an excellent appetite. The 81-year-old, wheelchair-bound man had lived with his 47-year-old son since being widowed 10 years earlier. He had multiple medical problems, including a below-the-knee amputation secondary to complications of diabetes. The son was employed as an evening-shift convenience store clerk and frequently stayed away from home two to three nights at a time. Mr. W. insisted that his son was a "good boy" and voiced no complaints about his care at home, but it was evident that he preferred not to elaborate. He refused to discuss the disposition of his monthly SSI check. An evaluation by the unit social worker revealed that the home was poorly kept and had virtually no foodstores. Attempts were made to engage the son in a more extended family evaluation and possible treatment, but he refused involvement. An application was filed for emergency Medicaid, and the patient returned home with a four-hour-per-day Medicaid-funded homemaker. He also began attending a three-day-per-week senior program, which provided transportation, and he received one meal daily from Meals on Wheels.

To prevent abusive situations from developing or worsening, great care should be taken to avoid high-risk discharge plans for elderly patients. The individuals who are to care for impaired elderly persons must be assessed, and, if they are found to be unsuitable, alternative care givers or placement may be necessary. Family therapy should be instituted where indicated.

Adult protective services exist in most states, and mandatory reporting of elder abuse is the law in many. Many criticisms have been leveled against both the protective services and the mandatory reporting laws, primarily as being ineffective and as infringements of patients' privacy and liberties (Reagan, 1985). Furthermore, designating all persons of a certain age to be in need of special protections may tend to stigmatize that age group.

Elder abuse is a complicated problem and defies easy solutions. Unfortunately, it is sure to exist as long as ageism and violence prevail (Kosberg, 1987). Psychiatrists and other mental health professionals must be alert to its signs, and be prepared to intervene, often by making alternative living arrangements for the patient upon discharge.

## RESEARCH AND THE ELDERLY PATIENT

If a competent inpatient consents to or refuses participation in a research protocol, it is the right of that patient to do so. As in treatment decisions, issues about the ability to consent to research participation arise only when the patient's competency is questioned. Here, again, it is important to consider competency to consent to research as decision specific; patients can be quite impaired but still capable, with proper explanation, of making a specific, competent decision about participation in a protocol. It is necessary that patients understand that they are being requested to participate in research, as well as the nature and consequences of participation in the research; that refusing to participate would not, in any way, jeopardize their care; and that the treatment they may (or may not) receive as part of the protocol is not intended primarily to be of benefit to them.

A patient's inclusion in a protocol and the stringency of the criteria used to evaluate the patient's understanding depend on the complexity and risk of the protocol. In minimal-risk protocols, every attempt should be made to tailor the consent information so as to increase the likelihood that even impaired individuals are able to participate in the consent process, reducing reliance on third-party representatives. A National Institute on Aging Task Force has developed advisory guidelines for research in senile dementia of the Alzheimer's type, which recommend that the consent of substituted decision makers be accepted for minimal-risk research, and for higher-risk protocols if they offer a realistic chance of benefit to the subject. If benefit is not likely, then specific approval by a judicial process would likely be required (Melnick, Dubler, & Weisbard, 1984). It is essential to work closely with one's own institutional review board to ensure that informed-consent procedures for the elderly conform to federal regulations.

## CONCLUSION

The elderly mentally ill are doubly compromised, subject to both the stigmatization that accrues to mental illness and the mistreatment and discrimination inherent in ageism. The delivery of quality care to the geriatric psychiatric patient requires the practitioner to address the patient's clinical needs without compromising autonomy and self-determination. This, in turn, requires knowledge of the special legal and ethical considerations raised in geriatric inpatient psychiatric treatment.

The clinician treating the geriatric psychiatric inpatient must be well versed in the clinical subtleties of competency assessment and be knowledgeable about the regulations bearing on informed consent, competency, and substituted judgment in his or her jurisdiction. This knowledge must be brought to bear on such issues as consent to hospitalization, civil commitment, consent to or refusal of psychotropic medications, and consent to ECT. Special attention must be paid to confidentiality, especially in relation to discharge planning with the patient's family. Of course, the clinician must be fully cognizant of all of the special clinical considerations that apply to the diagnosis, somatic treatment, and management of the geriatric patient in order to provide good care and to reduce the risk of liability. Special efforts must be made to preserve the patient's autonomy during discharge planning. Finally, the inpatient staff must have the capacity to refer the geriatric patient to appropriate social and legal services to facilitate such matters as long-term placement, health-care proxy, and estate planning.

## REFERENCES

American Psychiatric Association. (1983). Guidelines for legislation on the psychiatric hospitalization of adults. *American Journal of Psychiatry, 140,* 672–679.

Appelbaum, P. S., & Gutheil, T. G. (1982). *Clinical handbook of psychiatry and the law.* New York: McGraw-Hill.

Appelbaum, P., Mirkin, S., & Bateman, A. (1981). Empirical assessment of competency to consent to psychiatric hospitalization. *American Journal of Psychiatry, 138,* 1170–1176.

Appelbaum, P. S., & Roth, L. H. (1981). Clinical issues in the assessment of competency. *American Journal of Psychiatry, 138,* 1462–1467.

Baker, F. M., & Finkel, S. I. (1988). Legal issues in geriatric psychiatry. In L. Lazarus (Ed.), *Essentials of geriatric psychiatry* (p. 219). New York: Springer.

Barton, W. E., & Barton, G. M. (1983). *Mental health adminstration. Principles and practice* (Vol. 2). New York: Human Sciences Press.

Blank, K. (1987). Depressive illness in the elderly. In R. Rosner & H. I. Schwartz (Eds.), *Geriatric psychiatry and the law* (pp. 167–185). New York: Plenum.

Blank, K., Vingiano, W., & Schwartz, H. I. (1989). Psychiatric commitment of the elderly. *Journal of Geriatric Psychiatry and Neurology, 2,* 140–144.

Bluestone, H., Travin, S., & Kaufman, M. (1987). Administrative and forensic considerations in the operation of a geriatric psychiatry service. In R. Rosner & H. I. Schwartz (Eds.), *Geriatric psychiatry and the law* (pp. 205–239). New York: Plenum.

Brakel, J. B., Parry, J., & Weiner, B. A. (1985). *The mentally disabled and the law* (3d ed.). Chicago, IL: American Bar Foundation.

Chodoff, P. (1976). The case for involuntary hospitalization of the mentally ill. *American Journal of Psychiatry, 133,* 496–501.

Ciccone, R., & Clements, C. D. (1987). The elderly, incompetence, and treatment decisions: The New York experience. In R. Rosner & H. I. Schwartz (Eds.), *Geriatric psychiatry and the law* (pp. 29–48). New York: Plenum.

Dubler, N. N. (1988). Improving the discharge planning process: Distinguishing between coercion and choice. *Gerontologist, 28* (suppl.), 76–81.

Eth, S. (1991). Ethical issues in clinical care. In J. Sadavoy, L. W. Lazarus, & L. F. Jarvik (Eds.), *Comprehensive review of geriatric psychiatry* (pp. 653–666). Washington, DC: American Psychiatric Press.

Gardner, K., & Halamandaris, V. J. (1981). *Elder abuse (an examination of a hidden problem): A report with additional views by the Select Committee on Aging.* U.S. House of Representatives 87th Congress. Washington, DC: U.S. Government Printing Office.

Gaylin, W. (1982). The competence of children—no longer all or none. *Hastings Center Report, 12,* 33.

Goldstein, M. Z. (1989). Elder neglect, abuse and exploitation. In L. J. Dickstein & C. C. Nadelson (Eds.), *Family violence: Emerging issues of a national crisis* (pp. 99–124). Washington, DC: American Psychiatric Press.

Grossman, L., & Summers, F. (1980). A study of the capacity of schizophrenic patients to give informed consent. *Hospital and Community Psychiatry, 31,* 204–206.

Haug, M. (1979). Doctor-patient relationships and the older patient. *Journal of Gerontology, 34*(6), 852–860.

Jeste, D. V., & Wyatt, R. J. (1982). *Understanding and treating tardive dyskinesia.* New York: Guilford.

Jones, L. R., Parlour, R. R., & Badger, L. W. (1982). The inappropriate commitment of the aged. *Bulletin of the American Academy of Psychiatry and Law, 10,* 29–38.

Kapp, M. B., & Bigot, A. (1985). *Geriatrics and the law: Patient rights and professional responsibilities* (pp. 93–102). New York: Springer.

Kosberg, J. I. (1987). Abuse of the elderly: An overview of the problem and solutions. In R. Rosner & H. I. Schwartz (Eds.), *Geriatric psychiatry and the law* (pp. 241–257). New York: Plenum.

Kramer, B. A. (1987). Electroconvulsive therapy use in geriatric depression. *Journal of Nervous and Mental Disease, 175,* 233–235.

Meisel, A., Roth, L., & Lidz, C. (1977). Toward a model of the legal doctrine of informed consent. *American Journal of Psychiatry, 134,* 285–289.

Melnick, B. L., Dubler, N. N., & Weisbard, A. (1984). Clinical research in senile dementia of the Alzheimer's type: Suggested guidelines addressing the ethical and legal issues. *Journal of the American Geriatric Society, 32*(7), 531–536.

Miller, R. D. (1990a). Involuntary civil commitment. In R. I. Simon (Ed.), *Annual review of clinical psychiatry and the law.* Washington, DC: American Psychiatric Press.

Miller, R. D. (1990b). *Zinermon v. Burch:* No entrance? *Newsletter: American Academy of Psychiatry and the Law, 15,* 37–39.

Munetz, M. R., Kaufman, E. R., & Rich, C. L. (1980). Modernization of a mental health act: 1. Commitment patterns. *Bulletin of the American Academy of Psychiatry and Law, 8,* 83–93.

Okin, R. L. (1986). The relationship between legal status and patient characteristics in state hospitals. *American Journal of Psychiatry, 143,* 1233–1237.

Olin, G. B., & Olin, H. S. (1975). Informed consent in voluntary mental hospital admissions. *American Journal of Psychiatry, 132,* 938–941.

President's Commission for the Study of Ethical Problems in Medicine and Biomedical and Behavioral Research (1982). *Making health care decisions: The ethical and legal implications of informed consent in the patient–practitioner relationship.* Washington, DC: U.S. Government Printing Office.

Reagan, J. J. (1985). Protective services for the elderly: Benefit or threat. In J. I. Kosberg (Ed.), *Abuse and maltreatment of the elderly: Causes and interventions* (pp. 279–291). Boston, MA: Wright.

Ross, H. E., & Kedward, H. B. (1977). Psychogeriatric hospital admission from the community and institutions. *Journal of Gerontology, 32,* 420–427.

Roth, L. H. (1980). Mental health commitment: The state of the debate 1980. *Hospital and Community Psychiatry, 31,* 385–396.

Sadoff, R. L. (1991). Medical-legal issues. In J. Sadavoy, L. W. Lazarus, & L. F. Jarvik (Eds.), Comprehensive review of geriatric psychiatry (pp. 637–651). Washington, DC: American Psychiatric Press.

Saltz, B. L., Kane, J. M., Woerner, M. M., Lieberman, J. A., Alivir, J. M. J., Kahaner, K., & Foley, C. (1989). Prospective study of tardive dyskinesia in the elderly. *Psychopharmacology Bulletin, 25*(1), 52–56.

Salzman, C. (1984). *Clinical geriatric psychopharmacology.* New York: McGraw-Hill.

Schwartz, H. I., & Blank, K. (1986). Shifting competency during hospitalization: A model for informed consent decisions. *Hospital and Community Psychiatry, 37*(12), 1256–1260.

Schwartz, H. I., & Roth, L. H. (1989). Informed consent and competency in psychiatric practice. In A. Tasman (Ed.), *American Psychiatric Press review of psychiatry* (Vol. 8) (pp. 409–431). Washington, DC: American Psychiatric Press.

Schwitzgebel, R. I., & Schwitzgebel, R. K. (1980). *Law and psychological practice.* New York: Wiley.

Simon, R. I. (1987). Clinical psychiatry and the law (pp. 153–156). Washington, DC: American Psychiatric Press.

Smith, J. M., & Baldessarini, R. J. (1980). Changes in prevalence, severity and recovery in tardive dyskinesia with age. *Archives of General Psychiatry, 37,* 1368–1371.

Stanley, B., Stanley, M., & Pomara, N. (1985). Informed consent and geriatric patients. In B. Stanley (Ed.), *Geriatric psychiatry: Ethical and legal issues* (pp. 18–35). Washington, DC: American Psychiatric Press.

Stein, E. M. (1988). Normal aging—psychological and sociocultural aspects. In L. W. Lazarus (Ed.), *Essentials of geriatric psychiatry* (pp. 1–24). New York: Springer.

Strumpf, N. E., & Evans, L. K. (1988). Prolonged physical restraint: Promoting good vs. doing harm. Presented at Gerontological Society of America Annual Meeting, San Francisco, November 22.

Taub, H. A. (1980). Informed consent, memory and age. *Gerontologist, 20,* 686–690.

Tinetti, M. D., Liu, W. L., Marottoli, R. A., & Ginter, S. F. (1991). Mechanical restraint use among residents of skilled nursing facilities: Prevalence, patterns and predictors. *JAMA, 265,* 468–471.

Tomelleri, C. J., Lakshminawayanan, N., & Herjanic, M. (1977). Who are the committed? *Journal of Nervous and Mental Disease, 165,* 288–293.

Warheit, G. J., Longino, C. F., & Bradsher, J. E. (1991). Sociocultural aspects. In J. Sadavoy, L. W. Lazarus, & L. F. Jarvik (Eds.), *Comprehensive review of geriatric psychiatry* (pp. 99–116). Washington, DC: American Psychiatric Press.

Weiner, R. D. (1982). The role of electroconvulsive therapy in the treatment of depression in the elderly. *Journal of the American Geriatric Society, 30,* 710–712.

Winslade, W. J. (1988). Electroconvulsive therapy: Legal regulations, ethical concerns. *Review of psychiatry 1988* (Vol. 7). Washington, DC: American Psychiatric Press.

*Zinermon v. Burch,* 110 S.Ct. 975 (1990).

Zwerdling, I., Karasu, T., Plutchik, R., & Kellerman, S. (1975). A comparison of voluntary and involuntary patients in a state hospital. *American Journal of Orthopsychiatry, 45,* 81–97.

# 7

## Consultation–Liaison Psychiatry on the General Medical Wards

ROBERT WEINSTOCK AND
THOMAS GARRICK

The consultation liaison psychiatrist confers with staff members on medical and surgical wards who generally are not accustomed to treating patients with psychiatric disturbances. As such, many legal and ethical considerations involved in the treatment of psychiatric patients should be clarified for the medical team, including the nursing and social work staffs. The consulting psychiatrist must explain the extent to which psychiatric patients can be treated involuntarily, as well as the methods of obtaining authorization for medical and psychiatric treatment for incompetent patients. This chapter reviews the forensic issues commonly encountered by psychiatrists consulting to medical and surgical wards in a general hospital.

### DOCUMENTATION

Physicians have traditionally used the written record as a personal memory aid for following symptom evolution and treatment progress. However, pressure from many sources has transformed it into a public record that is used by insurers, utilization reviewers, quality assurance reviewers, investigative agencies, and attorneys. As part of the medical record, the written psychiatric consultation serves many purposes, not all of which directly relate to the clinical care of the patient (Garrick

& Stotland, 1982). While the usual psychiatric consultation is not written specifically for review, it may be used by reviewers at a later date for purposes not initially intended by the psychiatric consultant.

The written psychiatric consultation reflects the consultation–liaison psychiatrist's complex role in the medical-care system. The report is requested primarily as a physician-to-physician communication. However, by its very nature, it is also an official history and examination of the patient. It encompasses more than the physician's stated questions to the consultant, including as well many of the patient's expressed concerns. Although it does not constitute formal orders for nursing and support personnel in the care of the patient, it does provide a suggested management plan. Finally, it serves to document a specialist's opinion regarding the patient's care.

The psychiatric consultation must be written with these multiple purposes in mind (Garrick & Stotland, 1982). Although the report is expected to be as brief as possible in order to be read by the busy requesting physician, it must include all the pertinent information needed to support the diagnosis and recommendations, and provide adequate details as documentation of the patient's condition for future clinical and nonclinical (e.g., medicolegal) review (Hoffman, 1986). The language reflects these immediate audiences and purposes; it is a blend of medical and psychiatric terminology not usually intended for legal review.

The psychiatric consultant brings an important technical perspective to a medical and surgical treatment program. At the diagnostic end, the history and observation of mental-status changes often provide critical information about underlying biological and pathophysiological processes affecting the patient's bodily function. For example, a depressive syndrome may be a reflection of indolent thyroid dysfunction, new-onset brain disease (e.g., tumor, vasculitis, infection), metabolic dysfunction, or heart disease. The psychiatrist may identify idiosyncratic reactions to the treatment or disease process that put the patient at risk for treatment noncompliance. The psychiatric treatment may be integral to the patient's capacity to become involved in medical treatment. For example, management of depressive psychotic reactions may be crucial to a patient's capacity to consent to treatment. The medical treatment may cause disturbances in mental status that require psychiatric intervention, as in the case of steroid psychosis or beta-blocker–induced depressive syndromes. For these and other reasons, the psychiatric consultant's opinions are frequently central to the medical team's provision of safe and effective treatment (Stotland & Garrick, 1990).

It is, therefore, incumbent on the consulting psychiatrist to document adequately the history and mental-status examination. It is difficult to prove that certain observations, examinations, or interactions (e.g., informing the patient of potential adverse reactions to procedures or medicines) that were not documented were in fact performed. Similarly, consultees who request a psychiatric evaluation and ignore the findings or recommendations may place themselves at risk for liability for resulting damages to the patient. In certain situations, moreover, documentation alone may not be adequate; direct and immediate communication with the treating physician may be required, as in the case of emergencies or findings of critical importance to patient safety (*Merriman v. Toothaker,* 1973). Tactful documentation of such communications should be considered where liability is of concern. Some physicians fear that, when in doubt, uncertainties should not be documented in the medical record. In contrast, it is likely, in our opinion, that if there is doubt, it is especially important to include the logic behind a decision, including a risk–benefit analysis, since it demonstrates a reasoned process underlying the medical decision (Weinstock, Leong, & Silva, 1990). This documentation would at least show later reviewers that the decision was not a priori negligent, as might be the impression from an empty medical record. Explanations given after the fact that are not included in the record can be dismissed as self-serving. Actions should not be inconsistent with the documented record. If they are, it implies something is wrong either with the actions or the record.

## LIABILITY OF THE CONSULTANT AND CONSULTEE

Once the consultant is summoned, what is the extent of the consultant's responsibility for omissions or commissions? Although the published case law is scant in this area, malpractice insurers generally are familiar with actions directed at consultants to physicians. Most of these cases are settled out of court or do not reach the level of published court opinion. Despite the lack of published judicial opinion, consultants need to be aware of their own potential liability for injuries that may be associated with the clinical care—direct or indirect—provided by them.

The basis for consultant liability emanates from the consultant's special role in the health-care system. Legal authorities recognize that there are limits to the knowledge physicians can possess, and that they should not be held liable for information about a disease or drug outside of their expertise. It is for this reason that each physician is held to the standard of care common to other professionals of the practitioner's training and theoretical orientation (e.g., Appelbaum & Gutheil, 1991). The specialization of the medical-care system has led to the expectation that physicians will obtain consultation from suitable experts when confronting illnesses about which they are not professionally knowledgeable, and not hold themselves out as expert in areas in which they are not expert (e.g., Irwin, 1985; Prosser, 1971). Since the consultant is summoned by the primary treating physician, the consultant must provide such services with a degree of skill, knowledge, and care comparable to that of other psychiatrists working in the community (Prosser, 1971). To the extent that the standard of care is not met, the consultant could be liable for professional negligence.

There is a question as to whether the consultant has an independent duty to the patient or a duty solely to the primary physician. A physician generally must have a doctor–patient relationship before a breach of duty can be posited. It has been recognized in at least one jurisdiction that merely signing a prescription on behalf of another physician does not alone create a doctor–patient relationship (*Bass v. Barksdale,* 1984). Generally, the direct communication that occurs between physician consultant and patient, and the submission of a bill for services rendered, creates an independent physician–patient relationship (Irwin, 1985). To the extent that such a duty exists, any breach that is the proximate cause of damages to the patient could reasonably be actionable in a professional negligence claim. Consultants must use the same caution as when providing direct primary care to document and communicate findings, recommend reasonable diagnostic studies, and provide reasonable treatment recommendations. Thus the consultant's evaluation could be held to the same standard as that of the primary physician.

Most commonly, consultants are not in direct control of services provided to the patient. What is the consultant's responsibility for ensuring that the primary-care physician follows the recommendations? In some situations, the consultant becomes a treating physician along with the primary physician, and here the duties are clearer. However, more often, the consultant has been asked to give expert advice—not to take over treatment. In certain circumstances, the primary physician may consider the recommendations to be contraindicated to the patient's overall condition. For example, a cardiologist treating a depressed patient with advanced cardiac disease may choose not to use tricyclic antidepressants because of their potentially adverse cardiac effects, despite the psychiatric consultant's contrary opinion. Similarly, a rheumatologist treating a patient suffering from lupus arteritis with prednisone, that is causing a secondary psychosis, may believe it too dangerous to lower the steroid medications to alleviate the psychotic symptoms. Ordinarily, consultants would not report contrary opinions to the patient, but would leave communication of alternatives to the primary physician. At times, however, consultees choose not to follow recommendations because of ignorance, minimization of psychiatric problems, or uneasiness regarding psychiatric treatments.

Some legal authorities believe that once a consultant has been summoned, and has provided an opinion on a case, the consultee may have a duty to follow the advice, unless there is good reason not to do so (Prosser, 1971). For example, in *Largess v. Tatem* (1972), the Supreme Court of Vermont found a consultee negligent for failing to follow a consultant's recommendation to limit ambulation following orthopedic surgery and for failing to reconsult before recommending full physical activity. The apparent "indirect" nature of the consultant's relationship with the patient did not relieve the consultant of potential liability and responsibility toward the patient.

As noted, courts have determined that in certain situations the consultant has a direct duty to the patient (e.g., *Phillips v. Good Samaritan Hospital,* 1979). Where the consultant believes actual harm may come from the primary physician's actions, a definitive intervention could be necessary. At the very least, the consultant must provide reasonable and timely documentation of the recommendations. Case law is unclear as to whether the consultant merely has a duty to communicate adequately with the primary physician, or whether there also is a duty to communicate directly with the patient. There is also a question of whether and how much of a doctor–patient relationship exists independently for the consultant, or if it exists only indirectly through the primary physician.

Finally, what is the responsibility of the primary-care physician for the actions or recommendations of the consultant? Physicians (Irwin, 1985), legal commentators (Prosser, 1971), and case law (*Rise v. U.S.*, 1980) support the notion that a physician is expected to use ordinary, reasonable care in the selection of a competent consultant, and that a patient's consent is implied by his or her voluntarily accepting an evaluation by the consultant. When the care is turned over to the consultant, the liability of the referring physician ceases (*Jones v. Monte Fiore Hospital*, 1980). However, where the patient sustains damages as a result of the primary physician's following the consultant's advice, both physicians may be held liable under a theory of "joint venture" (Irwin, 1985) or "joint liability" (*O'Hara v. Architects*, 1975).

A joint venture is an association of two or more persons set up to carry out a single business enterprise for profit, for which purpose they combine their property and services. This theory was used successfully to sue a general practitioner who assisted a surgeon who left a drain in a patient (*Watts v. Jankowski*, 1980). Similarly, where the acts of two parties that alone may not have caused harm together result in damages to a third party, the two may be held jointly liable (Prosser, 1971). This is so because acts are not performed in isolation, but in the context of what others are doing; individuals are held accountable, to some extent, for acting in this context. Notably, however, the level of knowledge required by a primary general physician is not the same as that of a specialist. A primary physician may discharge his or her duty to the patient if he or she consults with a competent specialist, and if the level of knowledge required is beyond that ordinarily possessed by a primary physician. In such cases, it is likely that the consultant would be found liable if he or she were to provide negligent advice below the standard of care.

## PATIENTS WITHOUT CHOICES

Good Samaritan laws protect physicians from liability when providing "good faith" emergency care (e.g., Ladd, 1985) unless gross negligence occurs. In emergency situations, delirious patients can be treated without consent under the legal doctrine of implied consent (Fogel & Mills, 1986). Under English common law, it was recognized that a "reasonable person" would want to receive medical treatment in a true medical emergency even if impaired awareness precluded his or her giving consent. In nonemergency situations for patients clearly lacking the competence to give informed consent, there is substantial precedent for the physician's involving family members (e.g., *Bonner v. Moran*, 1941). The California courts, in dicta, have supported decision making by involved family members, and even have given guidelines for priorities involving different family members (*Barber v. Superior Court*, 1983). For example, an involved, but distant, family member should be given a greater role in surrogate decision making than a closer, uninvolved relative. A close significant other should be given a greater role than uninvolved family. In uncomplicated cases where the patient clearly lacks the capacity to give informed consent, many courts have encouraged physicians and the family to make decisions about medical treatment without involving the courts. However, if the procedure is risky, there is disagreement among family members, or there are indications that the patient would not have consented if competent, the case should be taken to court to avoid possible liability. A formal adjudication of competency should be undertaken with either a court order for treatment or appointment of a temporary guardian or conservator. In some states, courts designate a substitute decision maker, or make the decision themselves in nonemergency situations. It, therefore, is important to be aware of the relevant legal requirements in a particular state.

## INFORMED CONSENT

Although an assessment of a patient's capacity to give informed consent may be made by any physician, special knowledge of mental as well as medical facts puts the psychiatrist in the best position to consult on these cases. Psychiatrists sometimes avoid consulting on these issues, rationalizing that competency is a legal determination. However, most situations do not require a formal court adjudication of competency for medical procedures. The psychiatrist can have an opinion about competency or can use the term "capacity" to distinguish the determination from a formal judicial one. Many general psychiatrists probably try to avoid being consulted on these matters because of their own lack of clarity about or uneasiness regarding forensic and legal matters. Nonpsychiatric physicians, however, become uneasy about any necessity to assess a patient's mental state and have less expertise in the mental aspects of competence than a psychiatrist. Psychologists have less knowledge about the medical aspects.

In the 1970s, the standard for informed consent became patient-based. In *Canterbury v. Spence* (1972), the court held that a physician must disclose the information a "reasonable man" would need to make a treatment decision. The patient must be told if there is a potential for serious harm or death, and potential complications should be explained in understandable lay terms. Risks need not be disclosed, however, if their likelihood is negligible, and so knowledge of them is not necessary to help a "reasonable man" decide.

In the 1970s and 1980s, many states adopted relevant statutes to cope with patients who are not competent to give informed consent for medical treatment. In California, for example, mental health conservators may be appointed to consent to medical treatment for a patient, or the probate court may be petitioned to authorize treatment. Such authorization commonly is provided by appointing the medical staff as temporary medical conservators for an incompetent patient.

In current practice, informed consent requires (1) the provision of information, (2) that the patient be competent, and (3) that there be understanding (or appreciation) (Meisel, Roth, & Lidz, 1977). A precondition for a valid consent is that it be voluntary (free from unfair persuasion or inducements). Disclosure is needed and entails informing a patient of the risks, benefits, alternatives, and nature of treatment. States differ in their requirements as to what risks need to be presented to a patient. Some require only significant and substantial risks. Others do not require risks commonly known or those risks inherent in a procedure (Andrews, 1984). Exceptions to the need to get informed consent from a patient are (1) an emergency, (2) incompetency, (3) a waiver, and (4) therapeutic privilege. "Therapeutic privilege" (*Cobbs v. Grant,* 1972) has been referred to as the privilege to withhold information that would so upset a patient that he or she could not weigh it dispassionately. Since this privilege obviously can be subject to abuse, it is important to use it cautiously and with adequate documentation. The danger of patient upset needs to be substantially greater than average.

It is essential in assessing competency to give informed consent to remember that the average person will not function perfectly under the anxiety of a proposed medical procedure. Patients will be too anxious to think clearly. Casselith, Zupleis, and Sutton-Smith (1980), for example, found that only 60% of cancer patients tested one day after giving informed consent for chemotherapy, radiation, or surgery understood the nature and purpose of the treatment. Only 55% could list one potential complication, and only 40% read the forms carefully. Such deficits do not ordinarily make a patient incompetent unless they seriously interfere with the ability to weigh the risks and benefits of a procedure. To be declared incompetent to make a medical decision, a substantial deviation from the average is required.

## Tests for Competency to Give Informed Consent or to Refuse Consent for Medical and Psychiatric Treatment

In recent years, the subtler aspects of informed consent have received increasing attention in the literature. A consensus has been developing regarding certain basic aspects. Roth, Meisel, and Lidz (1977) proposed a threshold standard regarding tests for competency to consent to treatment based on the risks and benefits of a proposed treatment. If the risks were low and the benefits high, only the most basic test would be used for consenting patients. However, a very stringent test would be used for refusing patients in order to minimize the clear harm that refusal would ordinarily bring. If the risks were high and the benefits low, a stringent test would be used for consenting patients, but only a basic test for refusing patients. Weinstock (1986) expanded on this concept by endeavoring to arrive at an actual risk–benefit ratio to establish a threshold for competence. Estimates would be made of risks and benefits along a continuum and a ratio value obtained, rather than solely considering high and low risks and benefits as the only discrete categories. For example, there is a presumption with lifesaving, harmless procedures that a patient accepting such a procedure most likely is competent, but that a patient refusing it most likely is not. Similarly, with a risky experimental procedure of questionable benefit, there is a presumption that a patient refusing it is competent. If a patient were to accept, a stringent test would be used to ascertain that the patient fully understood and appreciated the risks. In between these two extreme examples, there is a continuum of test stringency or thresholds commensurate with varying risk–benefit ratios.

Similar concepts have been proposed by Drane (1984). Drane suggested a "sliding scale" model in which an increasingly more stringent standard would be utilized as the consequences of the patient's decision entailed more risk. Schwartz and Blank (1986) have called attention to the fact that the patient's clinical condition and the risks and benefits of a procedure shift during the course of treatment. They note the need to reassess patients continually and to keep in mind the concept of "partial competency," inasmuch as patients may be competent for some purposes, but not for others. Mahler and Perry (1988) point out that it may be permissible to withhold an opinion regarding competency until a psychiatric condition that is affecting competency is treated.

Spring and Winick (1991) propose utilizing sliding-scale standards based on variables pertinent to each individual patient. They make the point that since lawsuits based on the absence of informed consent are uncommon, the establishment of a trusting doctor–patient relationship that increases compliance and involves the patient in the decision-making process might be the most important rationale for informed consent. A 1982 Presidential Commission (see Andrews, 1984) concluded that capacity requires (1) the possession of a set of reasonably stable values and goals (but at certain outer limits, the goals may be so idiosyncratic as to call decision-making capacity into question); (2) the ability to communicate and to understand information; and (3) the ability to reason and deliberate about one's choices. It was recognized that decision-making capacity is specific to a particular decision, and is not dependent on the outcome per se, but on the patient's functioning in situations in which a decision about health care is to be made.

Appelbaum and Grisso (1988) have described a pragmatic set of functional criteria that may be utilized in assessing patients' competence to give informed consent. Patients must be able to (1) *communicate* their choice, (2) *understand* the relevant information, (3) *appreciate* the situation and the consequences of accepting or refusing treatment, and (4) *manipulate* the information of caretakers rationally. The first criterion is the most basic, and generally is the one utilized if there is no reason to question a patient's competency or if a minimum threshold is necessary. Ordinarily, there is an assumption of competence. The other criteria, in our opinion, should be applied in a more or a less stringent manner depending on the risks and benefits of a procedure, the resultant threshold for competence, and the ways in which deficits in these areas interfere with making a decision.

The second criterion is the one most often employed in competency assessments. An attempt is made to assess the degree of a patient's understanding. As stated by Weinstock (1986), more understanding is required when there is a higher threshold or a more stringent test of competency required based on the risk–benefit ratio. This criterion, therefore, should be applied with variable stringency dependent on the risk–benefit ratio. It is important, however, to ascertain that the information actually was supplied, and if necessary, to provide it again, perhaps with the primary physician present. Thorough understanding is not required, and in reality it is rarely achieved. It is not necessary that the patient know medicine. However, sufficient understanding is needed such that the risks and benefits can be weighed. For example, a high degree of understanding of a heart–lung transplant and its risks would be required if an unsuccessful operation would shorten a patient's life.

Appreciation includes acknowledging an illness, evaluating its effect and the effect of treatment options, and acknowledging the probabilities of risks and benefits. Problems can arise from pathological distortion or denial based on cognitive or affective impairment or the patient's delusional perceptions of his or her condition, the proposed treatment, or the motivations of caretakers. Denial of illness in some instances can prevent a competent decision. Since some denial of illness is usual, a marked lack of appreciation is necessary. A manifestly irrational decision, though not in and of itself a demonstration of incompetence, is a sign that the psychiatrist should look for impairment in the patient's capacity to weigh the risks and benefits. Lack of appreciation can be a possible explanation for a determination of incompetence, assuming that the patient has a cognitive understanding of the contemplated procedure.

Manipulating information rationally involves the thinking process and the weighing of information to reach a decision. A determination of incompetence is not based solely on outcome (that may, however, affect the threshold). It is based on the process, the chain of reasoning, or the way the decision is reached, not on the unconventional decision itself. A competent patient should be able to give "recognizable reasons" (Freedman, 1981), weigh the risks and benefits of options, and reach logically consistent conclusions. Reasoning may be compromised not only by psychotic thought disorders, delirium, and dementia affecting reasoning, but also by phobias, panic, anxiety, anger, depression, or euphoria. Although affective disorders sometimes lead only to deficits in "appreciation," cognitive disorders also can be present, such as an unrealistic view of the hopelessness of the situation.

If a patient cognitively understands a proposed procedure, an "irrational" decision alerts the psychiatrist to search for deficits in the consideration process in addition to "appreciation," since courts often have trouble understanding deficits solely in "appreciation." Alternatively, efforts should be made to try to understand how the decision makes sense from the patient's standpoint, considering the patient's values. An unconventional decision is not necessarily incompetent, even if the physician considers the decision ill advised. Patients who refuse treatment also should be giving "informed refusal" (*Truman v. Thomas,* 1980). Although criteria for assessing refusal generally are the same as for consent, patients need to be told, and need to understand and appreciate the risks of not following a recommended course of action. The physician's duty is to present to the patient all material risks a reasonable person would want to know about, including the risks of refusing, over and above the advantages of consenting.

In *Truman v. Thomas* (1980), a physician did not inform a patient that failure to get a Pap smear could lead to not detecting a possible cancer, and liability was found. Thus, informed refusal is also necessary.

A case example is that of a patient with mild paranoia but no other signs of an organic brain syndrome. His leg was developing gangrene and needed a below-the-knee amputation. This was an operation with risks (disfigurement), as well as benefits (saving his life). The patient's denial and suspiciousness were so strong, however, that he lost touch with reality. He refused to admit that his leg was getting worse. He, therefore, was considered by us not to be competent to refuse treatment. His family wanted the surgery, but were unwilling to override his wishes. The case was taken to court, and the judge appointed the hospital as temporary health-care conservator in order to pursue the treatment. After the operation, the patient was grateful and admitted he had been "out of it." Apparently, the gangrene had produced toxicity, even though no organic deficits were apparent on formal mental-status testing.

Brock and Wartman (1990) call attention to the need to be aware of irrational choices that competent patients often make, and to the need not to be too ready to declare patients making such choices incompetent. Examples of such irrational decision making are (1) bias toward the present and near future, ignoring distant harm; (2) an attitude of invulnerability and risk taking; (3) fear of pain or the medical experience; and (4) the ignoring of societal needs and irrational uses of resources. Such irrational factors operate in "normal" patients, and in most circumstances do not make them incompetent. Although Brock and Wartman include choices that do not make sense as also a "normal" phenomenon, a choice that is sufficiently irrational should motivate a psychiatrist to use the tests described in this chapter carefully, and to look for serious deficits in the thinking, appreciating, or understanding process that may be affecting competency and so may account for an irrational decision.

It is also important in assessing a patient's decision-making capacity to realize that the primary physician may not have given the patient an adequate explanation. The psychiatrist should explain the procedure again to the patient, perhaps with the primary physician present, before deciding that a patient lacks decision-making capacity. The psychiatrist's knowledge of the patient's psychodynamics and past history can be utilized, often with the assistance of family members and care givers more familiar to the patient, to change the patient's mind if he or she is making an unwise decision (Mahler & Perry, 1988).

For children and adolescents, consent of the custodial parent should be obtained. For emancipated minors, their own consent should be sufficient. For older adolescents, it is advisable to obtain consent from both parent and patient. Many states have specific laws that permit consent from an adolescent (e.g., birth control) in certain specified circumstances.

## REFUSAL OR WITHDRAWAL OF
## LIFE-SUSTAINING TREATMENT

Psychiatrists are sometimes involved in assessing a patient's capacity to refuse life-sustaining treatment. All hospitals receiving government funds are now required to provide all patients with information about advance directives (Omnibus Budget Reconciliation Act of 1990). Although patients are required to be competent in order to make such directives, criteria for its assessment are not specified. There has been recent continued attention in the courts to the issue of a patient's right to refuse life-sustaining treatment and the right to have a substitute decision maker make such a decision. In the case of *In re Quinlan* (1976), the New Jersey Supreme Court held that the patient's guardian or family would know best what her wishes would have been if she were able to consider her noncognitive vegetative existence. A "substituted judgment standard" was used in which the decision maker was expected to provide what the person herself would have decided if competent. Similarly, in *Superintendent v. Saikewicz* (1977), the Massachusetts Supreme Judicial Court utilized a substituted judgment standard, but required that an appointed guardian ad litem and the judge exercise the substituted judgment. In *In re Conroy* (1985), the New Jersey Supreme Court held that where clear evidence does not exist of what the person would have decided, an objective "best interest" standard may be applied. However, in situations in which family members do not act to protect a patient, the court needs to be on guard for abuse (*In re Jobes,* 1987).

California in the *Bouvia* case (*Bouvia v. Superior Court*, 1986) stated that a competent non-vegetative non-terminal patient with cerebral palsy and pain had a right to have tube feedings discontinued. Recently, the California Supreme Court (*Thor v. The Superior Court of Solano County*, 1993) extended this right to a prisoner who was quadriplegic, but was not in pain. The Court decided a competent person had the right to refuse nutrition or medication by feeding tube even if death would be the outcome of the decision. Although it would be reasonable to expect a fairly high threshold for competence to withhold life sustaining treatments unless the burdens of treatment were too great, the Court did not specify any criteria for competence.

Although distinctions have been made in some states between life-sustaining treatment and food and water, such a distinction was not made in a recent U.S. Supreme Court decision. In *Cruzan v. Director* (1990), Missouri required clear and convincing evidence of a patient's views before life-sustaining treatment could be terminated. The Supreme Court, in this decision, gave its first ruling on these issues. The Court held that a state's requirement that an incompetent patient's wishes as to the withdrawal of life-sustaining treatment be proven by clear and convincing evidence was not violative of due process.

In its decision, the majority of the Court clarified some important issues in these matters. As noted by Orentlicher (1990), the Court impliedly recognized a right under the U.S. Constitution to refuse medical treatment. The Court also found that a competent person can refuse life-sustaining hydration and nutrition, and that the right to refuse treatment survives a patient's incompetence and can be exercised by a substitute decision maker. However, states are permitted to differ in the procedural safeguards they employ to ensure that treatment withdrawal reflects a patient's wishes. Inferences from the decision are that the right to refuse medical treatment includes artificially supplied nutrition and hydration. The right is not limited to the terminally ill, and the right may be exercised through living wills, durable powers of attorney, or other advanced directives.

According to Orentlicher (1990), liability concerns should not deter an otherwise appropriate decision about terminating life-sustaining treatment. In fact, in California, courts have held that physicians could not be prosecuted for discontinuing life support systems, including feeding tubes, in accordance with patient or family instructions (*Barber v. Superior Court,* 1983) in cases in which the patient is not competent to make the decision. In contrast, refusal to honor a patient's request for withdrawing life support can in fact now lead to liability, as well as to costs for legal fees (*Bartling v. Glendale Medical Adventist Center,* 1986).

## Do Not Resuscitate Decisions

Psychiatrists may be asked to assess a patient's capacity to make a "Do Not Resuscitate" (DNR) decision. Similar considerations apply as with other instances of informed consent or refusal. In the future, it is possible that physicians may become involved in assisting the suicides of terminally ill patients or even in active euthanasia, in which the physician does the actual killing. This is an ethically complex area. Initially, only competent patients presumably would have this right of suicide. Some fear that this "right" would be extended, though, to surrogates in case of patient incompetence. Physicians would become killers, in contradiction to the Hippocratic Oath and medical tradition. Psychiatrists may then be asked to assess competence to make these decisions should such physician-assisted suicide or euthanasia become legal and ethically acceptable in the future.

Another controversial area involves situations in which medical staff members unilaterally make decisions to withhold treatment. In prior years, such decisions were made by unofficial "slow codes." These procedures can lead to liability because they ignore a patient's wishes and those of the family. More recently, some hospitals have adopted controversial policies of stating that resuscitation is not indicated for patients for whom staff members believe treatment is "futile." The American Medical Association (AMA) Council on Ethical and Judicial Affairs (1991) has called attention to the variability in physician definitions of "futile." "Futile has been variously interpreted as treatments with success rates ranging from 0 to 13%." The council cautioned that "these judgments of futility are appropriate only if the patient is the one to determine what is or is not of benefit, in keeping with his or her personal values or priorities." Although physicians can supply the medical evidence, they should not permit their personal value judgments about quality of life to obstruct the implementation of a patient's or surrogate's preferences regarding the use of cardiopulmonary resuscitation (CPR). If the physician determines that a treatment is medically futile in unusual circumstances, he or she can withhold CPR; however, the physician should, if time permits, inform the patient or surrogate and discuss alternatives so that a second opinion or transfer to another physician can be made.

According to Lo (1991), some patients could want treatment that would enable them to survive a few days even in a hospital. Perhaps they would wish to stay alive for a wedding, a graduation, or an anniversary, or to see a relative again. Value conflicts should not be confused with futility. Physiological futility such as an inability to restore cardiac function differs from quality of life or the inability to leave the hospital (Youngner, 1988); a persistent vegetative state also is different from severe disability. Since patients should be involved in DNR decisions, psychiatrists can be helpful in making sure that these issues are discussed compassionately. Physicians do a poor job of judging how patients view quality of life. They rated quality of life, physical comfort, mobility, depression, anxiety, and family relationships as significantly worse than did patients in one study (Ullmann & Pearlman, 1991).

Advance directives such as durable powers of attorney or living wills are important because substitute judgment makers do not always do a good job of knowing what a patient would have wanted—probably because of their own emotional reactions and the fact that families rarely discuss these issues beforehand. Physicians rarely know a patient's values. One recent study gives evidence of the poor ability to make substitute judgment decisions by both family and physicians (Suhl, Garrick, Reedy, & Sineous, 1990). Another study showed family members making decisions that were reasonably congruent with the patient's ideas, but not with the physician's (Seckler, Meier, Mulvill, & Paus, 1991). Advance directives should be encouraged to help avoid the problem of deciding and proving what a patient would have wanted if competent. Since these determinations can be quite difficult, perhaps impossible, advance directives need to be employed more often. Psychiatrists may be asked to assess patients' capacities to make decisions regarding advanced directives in questionable cases.

Patients may be competent to make decisions about DNR even if they are not competent for other medical purposes, or vice versa. Therefore, assessments of competency for the specific purpose are necessary despite the recent decision of the Supreme Court that for simplicity sake equated competence for one purpose with competence for another at least in the criminal arena (*Godinez v. Moran*, 1993). An illustrative case example is a 40-year-old, chronically schizophrenic woman who had a large duodenal adenocarcinoma and chronic renal failure and who refused dialysis because she was convinced that nothing was wrong with her kidneys despite what the doctors said. She was considered incompetent to make the decision because of her extreme denial and delusional belief that she was well and that the doctors were wrong. Her appreciation and reasoning were faulty despite her understanding of the dialysis procedure and cognitively knowing what the doctors had told her. Nevertheless, because her cooperation for dialysis was necessary, it was decided not to go to court. Beyond this, however, she said she wished DNR status because she wanted to be left alone if she ever became very ill, and she did not want thumping on her chest, tubes, or ventilators because of the discomfort she had endured for so long. She, therefore, was able to consider the risks and benefits of DNR (a medium threshold decision in these circumstances), and so was considered competent to make a DNR decision.

## CONFIDENTIALITY

Consulting psychiatrists need to share information with referring physicians. Sharing clinical information generally with a consultant directly involved in the care of a given patient does not need specific authorization if the patient has approved the referral. Similarly, there is no problem with sharing information with a referring physician unless the patient directs otherwise; letters of referral or replies to such letters require no specific authorization (American Psychiatric Association, 1987).

Psychiatrists consulting in a general hospital should be aware that information in a general medical record is not always as well protected as are psychiatric records. Information in a medical record should be limited to that which is necessary to meet the requirements of law and to maintain a documented database appropriate for continued treatment. The American Psychiatric Association (APA) guidelines (1987) recommend that "extraneous and irrelevant material should be kept to a minimum, as should material that is sensitive or potentially damaging to the patient or other persons."

There is no requirement for notifying family members or relatives about suicidal patients (see *Bellah v. Greenson,* 1978). However, it may be consistent with the standard of care to do so if there is reason to believe that the family might be helpful in preventing the suicide and there is no therapeutic contraindication to doing so. Legal worries about liability for violating confidentiality should not be important considerations since, according to Knapp and Van de Creek (1987), there is no court case in which a mental health professional has been successfully sued for violating confidentiality to protect a suicidal person. Liability, though, could be found for violating the profession's standard of care if measures are not taken to protect a suicidal patient. Notifying family or the people with whom the patient will be staying ordinarily might be required by the standard of care if a patient is not hospitalized, absent a good overriding reason not to violate confidentiality. Protection of life ordinarily should take precedence, however, and confidentiality maintained only if it is considered to be more protective of life.

Reporting laws not only can involve the consultant, but other medical staff members as well. Laws generally require reporting of child abuse, elder abuse, abuse of the developmentally disabled, and gunshot wounds. Reports may be required to the department of motor vehicles for patients with Alzheimer's disease and related dementias, and for patients potentially liable to suffer seizures or blackouts while driving. There also are requirements to report contagious diseases to public health officials and exposure to toxic chemicals in the workplace to state and federal agencies. Reporting of human immunodeficiency virus (HIV) status and notification of unknowing victims who may contract the virus from the patient are especially complex problems (Silva, Leong, Latz, & Weinstock, 1990), and requirements differ from state to state, necessitating familiarity by consultants with the local law. California currently also requires the reporting of all psychiatrically hospitalized patients even if voluntary, so that they can be prevented from purchasing a gun.

## TRANSFER AND RELOCATION

The transfer or release of patients who are dangerous to themselves, dangerous to others, or are unable to care for themselves may be a special problem in the general hospital. Ordinarily, discharge is determined by medical staff members, who solely consider stabilization of the acute medical condition and may ignore or miss any psychiatric issues. Such suits are common and can result in the largest judgments of all (Poythress, 1990). Psychiatrists are commonly consulted to assist in discharge placement for patients unable to care for themselves when these patients are considered to be medically stable. Requests for evaluation of "competency" at such points should be clarified in order to understand the real question. Such requests may represent a wish for an assessment of whether a patient can care for himself or herself or needs to be sent to a nursing home or psychiatric hospital, or may be merely an attempt to find a disposition. An assessment may be required of whether the patient meets the criteria for a conservatorship or guardianship. These assessments may be obtained through probate or mental health courts, and can be of the person and/or the estate. Guardianship may be necessary to send a patient to a nursing home against his or her wishes. Such assessments can prove difficult since they require that a patient be incompetent for most, if not all, legal purposes. Such global incompetence usually applies only in cases of severe dementia.

Since the psychiatrist observes the patient only in the hospital, it may prove difficult to extrapolate from the hospital to life circumstances outside. It may become necessary to consult with the family and nursing staff to obtain information relevant to a patient's functioning, in addition to the information obtained by a complete mental-status examination. The mental-status examination in such patients should focus on issues related to caring for oneself, such as calculating judgments regarding money, knowing how much things cost, and remembering recent information. Other methods of obtaining functional assessment might be considered, if feasible, such as home visits, direct observation of activities of daily living (ADL), or the use of functional assessment scales. Situations involving patients who are cognitively intact, but are physically unable to care for themselves, and are unwilling to enter a nursing home are particularly wrenching. In extreme situations, denial of physical illness may so interfere with a patient's ability to provide self-care as to limit his or her decision-making capabilities and so require a guardian or conservator.

Consultation with senior colleagues is the best way to show diligence (and lack of negligence). It even was encouraged in the Middle Ages, when a surgeon would be liable for money put up as bond only if the surgeon did not obtain consultation from a senior surgeon when there was a risk of loss of life or maiming (Cosman, 1982).

Physicians also can be held liable under the malpractice theory of "abandonment" (e.g., Halleck, 1980) if suitable arrangements for follow-up by the treating or another physician are not made. Physicians, including psychiatrists, have no duty to treat a patient they do not want to treat, and have no duty to prescribe a particular treatment a patient wants if the physician disagrees with the treatment. However, they do have a duty to make a suitable referral. Psychiatric consultants can be helpful in making other physicians aware of this requirement in cases in which they may wish to stop treating a patient who angers them too much. Physicians also can be made aware that they can refer a patient whom they dislike and do not wish to treat (especially in the private setting).

## CONSULTATION WITH HOSPITAL ATTORNEYS

Although hospital attorneys and risk management personnel can be helpful, they may place liability issues above a patient's welfare or psychiatric ethical considerations. The clinician should not defer clinical judgments to an attorney, but should discuss with the attorney how best to achieve clinical and ethical goals without incurring liability. Some physicians are overly concerned with imagined legal requirements or fears of liability in situations in which successful suits are unlikely. It has been recommended (McCrays & Wahman, 1990) that a disinterested legal advisor would provide a more objective, balanced appraisal of liability issues than would hospital counsel, by not ignoring the patient's welfare and preferences. However, it should be possible for a psychiatrist to discuss the case with the hospital attorney, with the realization that it is the clinician and not the attorney who makes the ultimate clinical decision. In problem situations, senior colleagues, hospital administrators, and hospital ethics committees should be consulted.

## REFERENCES

American Medical Association, Council on Ethical and Judicial Affairs. (1991). Guidelines for the appropriate use of Do Not Resuscitate orders. *JAMA, 265,* 1869–1871.

American Psychiatric Association. (1987). Guidelines on confidentiality. *American Journal of Psychiatry, 144,* 1522–1526.

Andrews, L. B. (1984). Informed consent statutes and the decision making process. *Journal of Legal Medicine, 5,* 196–197.

Appelbaum, P., & Grisso, T. (1988). Assessing patients' capacities to consent to treatment. *New England Journal of Medicine, 319,* 1635–1638.

Appelbaum, P., & Gutheil, T. (1991). *Clinical handbook of psychiatry and the law* (2d ed.). Baltimore, MD: Williams & Witkins.

*Barber v. Superior Court,* 147 Cal.App.3d 1006, 195 Cal.Rptr. 484 (1983).

*Bartling v. Glendale Medical Adventist Center,* 184 Cal.App.3d 961, 228 Cal.Rptr. 360 (1986).

*Bass v. Barksdale,* 671 SW2d 476 (Tenn. App. 1984).

*Bellah v. Greenson,* 81 Cal.App.3d 614, 146 Cal.Rptr. 535 (1978).

*Bonner v. Moran,* 126 F.2d 121 (D.C. Cir. 1941).

*Bouvia v. Superior Court,* 179 Cal.App.3d 1127, 225 Cal.Rptr. 297.

Brock, D., & Wartman, S. (1990). When competent patients make irrational choices. *New England Journal of Medicine, 322,* 1595–1599.

*Canterbury v. Spence,* 462 F.2d 772 (D.C. Cir. 1972).

Casselith, B., Zupleis, R., & Sutton-Smith, K. (1980). Informed consent: Why are its goals imperfectly realized? *New England Journal of Medicine, 302,* 896–900.

*Cobbs v. Grant,* 104 Cal.Rptr. 505, 8 Cal.3d 229 (1972).

Cosman, M. P. (1982). The medieval medical third party: Compulsory consultation and malpractice insurance. *Annals of Plastic Surgery, 8,* 152–162.

*Cruzan v. Director, Missouri Department of Health,* 110 S.Ct. 2841, 111 L.Ed.2d 224 (1990).

Drane, J. H. (1984). Competency to give informed consent: A model for making clinical assessments, *JAMA, 252,* 925–927.

Fogel, B. S., & Mills, M. J. (1986). Legal aspects of the treatment of delirium. *Hospital and Community Psychiatry, 37,* 154–158.

Freedman, B. (1981). Competence: Marginal and otherwise: Concepts and ethics. *International Journal of Law and Psychiatry, 4,* 53–72.

Garrick, T. R., & Stotland, N. L. (1982). How to write a psychiatric consultation. *American Journal of Psychiatry, 139,* 849–855.

*Godinez v. Moran,* 113 S.Ct. 2680 (1993).

Halleck, S. (1980). *Law in the practice of psychiatry.* New York: Plenum.

Hoffman, B. F. (1986). How to write a psychiatric report for litigation following a personal injury. *American Journal of Psychiatry, 143,* 164–169.

*In re Conroy,* 98 N.J. 361, 486 A.2d 1229 (1985).

*In re Jobes,* 108 N.J. 394, 529 A.2d 434 (1987).

*In re Quinlan,* 40 N.J. 10, 355 A.2d 47, *cert. denied,* 429 U.S. 922 (1976).

Irwin, J. R. (1985). Legal implications of intraoperative consultation. *Urologic Clinics of North America, 12,* 557–570.

*Jones v. Monte Fiore Hospital,* 418 A. 2d. 1361 (Pa.Super. 1980).

Knapp, S., & Van de Creek, L. (1987). *Privileged communication in the mental health professions.* New York: Van Nostrand Reinhold.

Ladd, R. E. (1985). Patients without choices: The ethics of decision making in emergency medicine. *Journal of Emergency Medicine, 3,* 149–156.

*Largess v. Tatum,* 130 Vt. 271, 291 A.2d 398 (1972).

Lo, B. (1991). Unanswered questions about DNR orders. *JAMA, 265,* 1874–1875.

Mahler, J., & Perry, S. (1988). Assessing competency in the physically ill: Guidelines for psychiatric consultants. *Hospital and Community Psychiatry, 37,* 856–861.

McCrays, V., & Wahman, A. T. (1990). Procedural paternalism in competency determination. *Law, Medicine and Health Care, 18,* 108–113.

Meisel, A., Roth, L., & Lidz, C. (1977). Toward a model of the legal doctrine of informed consent. *American Journal of Psychiatry, 134,* 285.

*Merriman v. Toothaker,* 9 Wash.App. 810, 515 P. 2d 509 (1973).

*O'Hara v. Architects Hartung and Associates,* 326 N.E.2d 283 (Ind.App. 1975).

Orentlicher, D. (1990). The right to die after *Cruzan. JAMA, 264,* 444–446.

*Phillips v. Good Samaritan Hospital,* 65 Ohio App.2d 112, 416 N.E.2d 646 (1979).

Poythress, N. G. (1990). Avoiding negligent release: Contemporary clinical and risk management strategies. *American Journal of Psychiatry, 147,* 994–997.

Prosser, W. (1971). *Negligence.* St. Paul, MN: West.

*Rise v. U.S.,* 630 F.2d 1068 (5th Cir. 1980).

Roth, L., Meisel, A., & Lidz, C. (1977). Tests of competency to consent to treatment. *American Journal of Psychiatry, 134,* 279–284.

Schwartz, A., & Blank, K. (1986). Shifting competency during hospitalization: A model for reformed consent decisions. *Hospital and Community Psychiatry, 37,* 1256–1260.

Seckler, A. B., Meier, D. E., Mulvill, M., & Paus, B. E. (1991). Substituted judgment: How accurate are proxy predictions? *Annals of Internal Medicine, 115,* 92–98.

Silva, J. A., Leong, G., Latz, S., & Weinstock, R. (1990). Confidentiality in the era of AIDS. In R. Simon (Ed.), *Review of clinical psychiatry and the law* (Vol. 1). Washington, DC: American Psychiatric Press.

Spring, C., & Winick, B. (1991). Informed consent in theory and practice: Legal and medical perspectives on the informed consent doctrine and a proposed reconceptualization. *Critical Care Medicine, 17,* 1346–1354.

Stotland, N., & Garrick, T. (1990). *Manual of psychiatric consultation.* Washington, DC: American Psychiatric Press.

Suhl, J., Garrick, T., Reedy, T., & Sineous, P. (1990). Choices of patients and their surrogates regarding life support. *Proceedings of the 37th Annual Meeting of the Academy of Psychosomatic Medicine, 29.*

*Superintendent of Belchertown State School v. Saikewicz,* 373 Mass. 728, 370 N.E.2d 417 (1977).

*Thor v. The Superior Court of Solano County,* 93 Daily Journal D.A.R. 9579 (1993).

*Truman v. Thomas,* 27 Cal.3d 285 (1980).

Ullmann, R. F., & Pearlman, R. A. (1991). Perceived quality of life and preferences for life-sustaining treatment in older adults. *Archives of Internal Medicine, 151,* 495–497.

*Watts v. Jankowski,* 411 N.E.2d 678 (Ind.App. 1980).

Weinstock, R. (1986). Informed consent and competence issues in the elderly. In R. Rosner & H. Schwartz (Eds.), *Geriatric psychiatry and the law* (pp. 49–78). New York: Plenum.

Weinstock, R., Leong, G. B., & Silva, J. A. (1990). Confidentiality and privilege. In R. Simon (Ed.), *Review of clinical psychiatry and the law* (Vol. 1). Washington, DC: American Psychiatric Press.

Youngner, S. J. (1988). Who defines futility? *JAMA, 260,* 2094–2095.

# PART III
# Outpatient Services

# 8

# Forensic Problems Encountered in the Practice of Child and Adolescent Psychiatry

RICARDO M. VELA,
JOSÉ ARTURO SANCHEZ-LACAY, AND
HARVEY BLUESTONE

Want it or not, the child and adolescent psychiatrist inevitably gets drawn into dealing with forensic problems in the course of his or her practice. This is due, in part, to the increasing litigiousness that threatens psychiatric practice, the explosive expansion of rules and regulations controlling service delivery, and the increasing demands for accountability for actions taken in the rendition of services.

As stated by Robson (1992), the child and adolescent psychiatrist must be able to utilize and master both clinical and forensic knowledge to be competent in the field. Books and articles on forensic psychiatry provide some general principles and current trends of thinking based on previous court decisions. In reality, however, owing to the complexities and peculiarities of each individual case, there frequently are no clear guidelines to be followed. Forensic problems that arise in the practice of child and adolescent psychiatry thus are an uncharted challenge. Nevertheless, this state of affairs does leave some room for the creative and conscientious resolution of forensic problems. Above all, the principle of acting in the best interest of the child or adolescent and the principle of avoiding harm as much as possible must prevail in every decision that the psychiatrist makes.

This chapter does not attempt to deal with the forensic issues with which the child and adolescent psychiatrist voluntarily becomes involved, such as child custody evaluations, civil litigation, and the provision of expert testimony. Instead, it focuses on issues related to the interface between psychiatry and the law encountered in the course of the everyday practice of child and adolescent psychiatry. As stated by Schetky (1992), the child and adolescent psychiatrist should not be intimidated by the legal system or the possibility of malpractice litigation. Each case that involves forensic issues inevitably will result in a learning experience. It is in this light that the following five cases are presented. The cases are sample vignettes that were gathered from the authors' practices or supervision of child and adolescent psychiatry in a general hospital.

## CASE VIGNETTES

### Case 1: The Litigious Mother

Sam, a 15-year-old adolescent boy, came to the clinic accompanied by his mother, who stated she did not agree with the State Committee on Special Education's recommendations for special class placement and wanted a second opinion from the child and adolescent psychiatrist. Sam's mother, an angry, demanding woman, with an exaggerated sense of entitlement and evident paranoid and narcissistic traits, had turned the child over to the state social service authorities several years previously. Sam first was put in foster placement with his grandparents, but was later transferred to a group home, where he allegedly had been raped. Since that incident, the child had become suspicious, guarded, and mistrusting of adults. At the time of the clinic visit, the mother had regained custody of the child and had initiated a lawsuit against the group home.

The Committee on Special Education had initially classified Sam as "educable mentally retarded," and he was placed accordingly. Episodes of aggressive behavior, resulting from other students' provocations in the classroom, prompted a psychosocial reevaluation. The evaluation elicited a history of hallucinations in an uncooperative child who behaved inappropriately during the testing session. He was reclassified as "emotionally disturbed." Sam's mother disagreed with the recommendations. She had visited a long list of schools that the Committee on Special Education had recommended and was not satisfied with any of them. She demanded that the child be placed in a "quiet" private school based on the fact that, by state law, the Committee on Special Education must pay for a private school program if it is unable to find an appropriate school placement. Sam's mother did not accept the fact that he was mentally retarded, although psychological testing had assessed Sam's I.Q. at 57. She had consulted a lawyer, who asserted that an I.Q. score by itself, without an assessment of functioning, was not sufficient to make the diagnosis of mental retardation. She claimed that the evaluation had omitted such an assessment. In addition, she indignantly proclaimed that the label "mentally retarded" would be damaging to her child. She wanted the psychiatrist to write a letter supporting her claim.

Mental examination by the child and adolescent psychiatrist revealed limitations in multiple cognitive areas in an adolescent who was uncooperative and paranoid. Several sessions were required in order to allow Sam's mother to ventilate her feelings. She discussed her fears of having her child labeled "retarded" and entrapped in the bureaucratic system. Through empathic support and upon having the nature of the diagnosis clarified for her, the mother was able to accept the reality of her son's mental retardation. She agreed that it would be in his best interest to attend a class for the mentally retarded where more educational resources would be available. She then returned to the Committee on Special Education, where she negotiated a compromise whereby Sam would be kept in a class for the mentally retarded, but would be transferred to a classroom with less provoking and less aggressive children. A complicated futile legal process was thus avoided.

## Discussion of Case 1

This case is an example of the child and adolescent psychiatrist's acting as a "de facto magistrate" (see Chapter 1). State courts and legislatures have, in practice, failed to define substantive rights, deferring to the judgment of health practitioners. The reasoning behind this reluctance of the courts to be more specific in their definitions is that neither judges nor administrative hearing officers are better qualified than a psychiatrist to make psychiatric determinations. This state of affairs places a great deal of responsibility on the child and adolescent psychiatrist, who must take special care in making conscientious and sound recommendations in his or her role as a de facto magistrate.

Sam's mother asked for a second opinion from the clinic psychiatrist because of her disagreement with the determination of a public education agency about the child's class placement. Fortunately for all parties involved, the psychiatrist enabled Sam's mother to ventilate her anger and express her concern. Parental counseling provided the mother with information that ultimately resulted in her acceptance of the recommendations of the Committee on Special Education. Had she not accepted the psychiatrist's opinion and gone to court for a hearing on her plea, it would have been extremely unlikely that the court would have ruled against the qualified psychiatrist's expert opinion. Of course, Sam's mother would have been free not to use the services of her catchment area general hospital clinic and to get another independent psychiatrist to agree with her original position. But even if a private psychiatrist were available and willing, Sam's mother would not have the resources to pay for the evaluation, written reports, or the psychiatrist's court appearance. (If she were more affluent, she could have bypassed the public school system and placed the child in a private school for children with special needs.)

Child and adolescent psychiatrists working in clinics for indigent populations have, therefore, great power in their clinical decision making regarding potential forensic cases. This puts an extraordinary amount of responsibility on the psychiatrist and demands that he or she be very scrupulous, honest, and objective in exercising the most careful clinical judgment to make the right assessment. The community or general hospital clinic may provide a forum for case discussion or professional consultation when there is any doubt about making a recommendation with important implications. Above all, it is most important not to misuse the law and the power it has conferred on psychiatrists as de facto magistrates.

## Case 2: Persistent Refusal of Treatment

Roberto, a 13-year-old boy, was referred by the school counselor to the Child and Adolescent Crisis Team because of suicidal behavior.

The day before the referral was made, Roberto had locked himself in the bathroom and put a knife to his chest with the intention of stabbing himself. He came to the clinic accompanied by his mother. When examined by the clinic child and adolescent psychiatrist, Roberto complained that other kids at school fought him, kicked him in the stomach, and took his lunch money. He said that if his classmates were to beat him again, he would kill himself. The psychiatrist elicited a history of depression of two months' duration and of difficulty in sleeping. Roberto was assessed as being at high suicidal risk and referred to the state children's psychiatric hospital for inpatient treatment. After the child and adolescent psychiatrist discussed his findings and worked through Roberto's mother's denial and externalization of problems, the mother reluctantly accepted the referral for psychiatric hospitalization.

The psychiatrist who examined the child at the hospital determined that Roberto was indeed depressed, but, in his assessment, he minimized the risk of suicidality. He did not deem admission necessary, but strongly recommended to the mother that Roberto should receive treatment in the form of crisis intervention. Roberto's mother, who suffered from a severe borderline personality disorder with frequent angry outbursts, poor impulse control, and excessive use of splitting as a defense mechanism, refused the recommended treatment. The hospital psychiatrist reported Roberto's mother to the child protection agency for lack of compliance with medical treatment.

The child protection agency put pressure on Roberto's mother to bring the child back to the clinic. When seen with her child four days later, a very angry, uncooperative, indignant mother refused to reason with the crisis team nurse and instead denied that her son had any psychiatric problems. She rambled on about how people were unfairly blaming her for her son's problems. Roberto sided with his mother, denying his psychiatric symptoms, refusing treatment, and saying that he did not want to cause his mother any more problems. Before leaving the clinic, the patient's mother apologized for her angry behavior, but refused a follow-up appointment.

The state child protection agency was again informed of Roberto's mother's refusal of treatment. The case was taken to court, where a judge ordered outpatient treatment for Roberto. The mother returned to the crisis team. She was verbally abusive to the nurse and stated angrily that she had "no time to waste coming to the clinic," and that her son had a learning problem, but no major psychiatric illness.

When examined by the clinic child and adolescent psychiatrist, Roberto was minimally cooperative, suspicious, and guarded. He admitted to having had suicidal ideation in the past month, but denied being suicidal or homicidal at the moment. Nevertheless, he reported crowding of thoughts and delusions of thought insertion, indicating a psychotic process. Treatment with psychotropic medication was recommended, and again Roberto's mother went into an uproar, refusing any kind of treatment.

Roberto's mother was reported for a third time to the state child protection agency for medical neglect. The court order for psychiatric treatment was reinforced, and seven weeks later, Roberto was back in the clinic with his mother. The child and adolescent psychiatrist reexamined the child. At this time, Roberto denied any hallucinations, thought insertion, or withdrawal. The youngster showed signs of better interpersonal relatedness during the mental-status examination. He reportedly had been doing better in school.

The psychiatrist felt it would be best not to insist on prescribing psychotropic medication at the time, but that, instead, the child should come to weekly therapy sessions, during which the presence of psychotic symptoms or suicidal ideation would be assessed. If it became necessary, medication would be instituted. The treatment plan was discussed with Roberto's mother, who agreed to it. She requested that the child and adolescent psychiatrist send a letter to the child protection agency indicating her compliance with the treatment.

### Discussion of Case 2

Legal standards regarding children and adolescents' commitment to inpatient facilities have historically taken different courses. In the past, children were subjected to the doctrine of *parens patriae,* whereby they had no legal rights and decisions about their welfare were made by their parents, guardians, or the State. In the 1960s, the U.S. Supreme Court (*In re Gault,* 1967) held that the doctrine of *parens patriae* had been unconstitutionally applied, mandating due-process requirements and other procedural protections (Burlingame & Amaya, 1992; Kalogerakis, 1992). Later, the Supreme Court reversed its earlier trend and left intact state statutes that authorized parents and guardians to consent to psychiatric admissions. The court did not mandate judicial or administrative review, but determined that some kind of inquiry should be made by a "neutral fact finder" to determine whether the statutory requirements for admissions were satisfied (*Parham v. J.R.*, 1979).

At present, state approaches to the issue of involuntary admissions of children and adolescents are diverse and constantly changing. The issue of mandated outpatient treatment is an even less charted area. In some states, a presiding judge may order "outpatient commitment" when this is recommended by a psychiatrist. Involuntary outpatient commitment may be ordered by a court (1) as a conditional release from inpatient hospitalization, (2) based on less stringent criteria than for inpatient commitment, or (3) as a less restrictive alternative for persons who would meet the criteria for hospitalization but could benefit from community treatment. The failure to attend sessions may result in the return of a minor to an inpatient setting (Burlingame & Amaya, 1992).

In this case, inpatient admission would have proceeded without complications if the psychiatrist at the state institution had hospitalized the child. Outpatient treatment became more difficult to implement. This was complicated by the oscillating personality psychopathology of the patient's mother. The outpatient psychiatrist was caught between two conflicting forensic issues: the duty to protect and the patient's (and parent's) right to refuse treatment. The psychiatrist's judgment was that patient protection overrode the mother's right to refuse treatment. The psychiatrist was able to utilize the collaboration of the child protection agency to insist on treatment for this high-risk suicidal adolescent patient.

The child protection agency took the initiative of requesting the procedure of "outpatient commitment" from the court. This empowered the psychiatrist to overcome the recalcitrant mother's obstacles to treatment and to act in the best interest of the child.

## Case 3: "Doctor, please don't tell my parents"
Jane, a 14-year-old female living with her mother, stepfather, 18-year-old stepbrother, and three younger siblings, was brought to the emergency room of an inner-city general hospital following a suicide

attempt with an overdose of an over-the-counter medication. The patient was treated in the emergency room and admitted to the adolescent medical unit. A pregnancy test, done as part of the routine admissions laboratory workup, was positive. When questioned, Jane alleged that she had been raped by a "school friend." Further inquiry was able to elicit only very vague and contradictory responses in terms of the identity of the perpetrator, the location of the incident, and other circumstances related to the alleged rape, giving the impression that the patient was trying to conceal important information.

The pediatric consultation/liaison child and adolescent psychiatrist was asked to assess the patient's suicide potential and the alleged rape incident. Psychiatric examination revealed a depressed, guarded, marginally cooperative adolescent who would provide only minimal information in answer to the interviewer's questions. When confronted about her guardedness, the patient expressed fear that disclosure of her pregnancy to her parents would result in punishment. She begged the psychiatrist to keep the information confidential. Nevertheless, the psychiatrist was firm in his assessment that, in this case, the issue of confidentiality was overriden by the legal obligation to protect the minor. At a meeting of the attending pediatrician, pediatric house staff, the unit social worker, and the psychiatrist, the decision was made to inform Jane's parents of her pregnancy and to report the case to the child protection agency.

Because of her allegations of being raped by a nonfamily member, the child protection agency involved the police sex crime unit in the investigation. Suspicion that Jane's adult stepbrother might be the perpetrator, based on his behavior during visiting hours, prompted a police interrogation. He admitted to his sexual involvement with the patient.

Both the patient and her parents were informed in separate interviews about the alternatives available to deal with the pregnancy. Jane's parents, who were profoundly ashamed and enraged, immediately requested an abortion, but Jane, supported by her stepbrother, refused to consent to the procedure. A conflict thus ensued. Nevertheless, the parents succeeded in convincing Jane's stepbrother of the advisability of the abortion in view of the social stigma that completion of the pregnancy would bring. With the loss of her stepbrother's support, Jane had second thoughts about her desire to have the baby and requested an abortion. The abortion was performed, and Jane's parents pressed charges against her stepbrother. He pleaded guilty and was sentenced to community service. He was removed from the home and went to live with other relatives.

## Discussion of Case 3

There are three forensic principles that interplay in Jane's case: (1) confidentiality, (2) consent to treatment, and (3) the duty of the psychiatrist to protect the minor. In general, unless otherwise stipulated by statute, it may be assumed that a parent is legally entitled not only to authorize the treatment of a minor, but also to receive information about treatment, including any confidential information revealed by the adolescent (Macbeth, 1992). In the case of certain types of health care, including prenatal care, abortion, and birth control, however, minor-treatment statutes entitle the adolescent to care without parental knowledge (Kriechman, 1989). Confidentiality rules generally bar the disclosure of any information learned from the patient to any person not directly involved in the current patient care (Macbeth, 1992).

Nevertheless, as noted by Appelbaum and Gutheil (1991), confidentiality is not an absolute principle, and, in the face of countervailing duties, it may have to be overriden. This is the case with child physical or sexual abuse. In all jurisdictions in the United States, physicians are required by law to report cases of child abuse and sexual abuse. In most jurisdictions, the duty of a physician to report the abuse of a minor overrides the confidentiality rules. In fact, physicians who do not report abuse cases may be subject to criminal penalties, fines, and even imprisonment (Benedek, 1992).

In this case, in view of the child and adolescent psychiatrist's overriding duty to report the sexual abuse to the child protective authorities, Jane's request to keep the information confidential could not be granted. In all practicality, it would have been impossible to keep the information about Jane's pregnancy from her parents since the child protection agency had the obligation to investigate the case with the patient's family.

This still did not resolve the issue of who would be the indicated person to give consent for an abortion. Initially, Jane refused the procedure, a decision that was in direct conflict with the views of her parents. Notwithstanding, as explained in the next section, under New York State law, parental consent for treatment is not required for performing an abortion. Therefore, in this case, the patient had the last word in deciding whether she wanted to terminate pregnancy or carry the child to term. In addition, Jane was protected from further sexual abuse by the removal of her stepbrother from the home.

## Case 4: The Parents Were Not Told

Blanca, a 15-year-old adolescent female, was admitted to the adolescent medical ward of a general hospital following a suicide attempt. A few days before her admission, the patient had learned that she was pregnant. A heated argument ensued after Blanca's boyfriend, who was responsible for the pregnancy, strongly objected to the idea of Blanca's carrying the pregnancy to term. As a result, she became dysphoric and felt what seemed unbearable stress. She did not inform her parents about her pregnancy. Blanca planned her suicide, bidding farewell to her friends and boyfriend, and waiting to be alone in the house to carry out her plan. After ingesting more than 30 aspirin tablets, she was found in her bed the next morning in a semicomatose state. She was admitted to the intensive care unit, where she remained unconscious for two days. A pregnancy test confirmed that Blanca was indeed pregnant, and a sonogram assessed the gestational age as less than 12 weeks. The patient was told that, as a result of the toxicity of the aspirin, the health of the fetus was probably compromised. Blanca made the decision on her own to have an abortion, and she asked the medical staff not to inform her parents about her pregnancy or the abortion. The child and adolescent psychiatrist was called to consult about the patient's suicidality and to give an opinion as to whether Blanca's parents had to be notified or had to consent to treatment. The abortion proceeded without either parental notification or consent. The patient's ability to give her consent independently helped to change her passive helplessness and allowed her to assume more control of her life situation.

### Discussion of Case 4

Treatment without parental consent is allowed in four major circumstances: (1) in emergencies, (2) for emancipated minors, (3) for "mature" minors, and (4) according to specific consent statutes (Kriechman, 1989; Macbeth, 1992). Although this did not happen, this adolescent could have been treated for her drug intoxification, even if the parents could not be located to give consent, based on the emergency nature of her condition. Specific consent statutes in many states grant special rights to teenagers for confidential advice on contraception and the treatment of pregnancy-related conditions. In New York State, adolescents may consent to confidential abortion without the need of parental consent or disclosure. Therefore, in contrast to the previous case, this youngster's plea for confidentiality was backed by statute-mandated silence.

As an extra note of interest, the status of "emancipated minor," which would also enable the patient to obtain treatment without parental consent, may be awarded in certain jurisdictions to pregnant adolescents. Nevertheless, some states require that a court be petitioned and a court order of emancipation be obtained before medical treatment can begin (Kriechman, 1989). The court may decide to grant or reject an emancipation status on the basis of such factors as economic independence, general adult consent, and freedom from the control of parents (Macbeth, 1992).

## Case 5: The Anonymous Emergency Telephone Call

Susan, an 11½-year-old girl, had been in therapy at the clinic for over a year. She was initially referred by her school because of her excessively demanding behavior with the teacher, a lack of friends, an inability to get along with her peers, and her aggressive and provocative behavior. The child had feelings of being rejected by her mother and friends and could not tolerate sharing her teacher with the rest of the students unless given special one-to-one attention. She had been diagnosed as having a borderline (personality) disorder of childhood.

As Susan's relationship with the therapist intensified, she started transgressing the limits of therapy. Periods of demanding behavior alternated with clingingness at some times and angry outbursts at others. Her intense separation anxiety would lead to episodes of emotional instability and disorganization toward the end of a therapy session. On one occasion, she verbalized her ambivalent feelings about and confusion between her intense primitive wish for closeness and her fear of being smothered and engulfed by saying, "I wish you were an octopus and swallowed me and choked me to death." On other occasions, the child pretended during play sessions to report the therapist to the police for mistreating her.

As time went by, material from the sessions began to go beyond the therapy hour and the therapeutic relationship. Susan managed to get the therapist's telephone number and address, and she started leaving messages on his answering machine. When the therapist announced that he was terminating his job, and hence her therapy, the intensity of Susan's anxiety, anger, and feelings of rejection deepened. On one occasion, the therapist received a visit from the police in answer to a report to 911 that a burglary was in progress at his apartment. A month later, two calls were made to 911 during the same night—the first reporting a fire in the therapist's home, and the second that an infant there was in cardiac arrest. The latter brought the immediate attention of emergency medical services to the puzzled therapist's apartment.

The therapist strongly suspected that Susan had made the emergency telephone calls, but had no proof. When asked, the patient denied ever calling the police. At this point, the therapist faced the following dilemma. He did not have solid grounds on which to confront the patient with her disruptive acting-out behavior. On the other hand, he felt that therapy could not continue if this issue were not discussed. It needed to be managed therapeutically and limits set on the child's behavior.

Following a case conference at the clinic, it was decided that the therapist would formally file a complaint with the police. This allowed him to listen to the 911 recordings that had reported the alleged emergencies and he was able to identify the girl's voice. He thus was enabled to confront Susan with the confirmed behavior. She was told that if a similar incident occurred again, therapy would be stopped and only emergency services would be provided by the clinic. No charges were pressed. The patient never called the therapist's home or the police again, and therapy was terminated as scheduled.

## Discussion of Case 5

This case illustrates some of the difficulties encountered in treating a severely disturbed patient who transgresses the boundaries of therapy to involve the therapist in actions that can have potentially serious repercussions. The moment a clinician enters a relationship with a patient, a legal relationship also arises. It is naive, in our litigious society, to ignore the legal aspects of the therapeutic relationship. In most cases, the working alliance will develop and terminate without legal upheavals, but there is always the potential for it to end in legal complications.

In this case, the patient's intense attachment to the therapist resulted in the involvement of public health and law enforcement institutions. Not only was there the unlawfulness of falsely reporting a problem requiring the immediate mobilization of emergency medical services, but also the potential for depriving a seriously ill individual of prompt lifesaving medical attention while the service was responding to the false report.

Upon the child's denial of her actions, the therapist was confronted with the conflict between the legal situation and his duty to maintain a therapeutic relationship and provide treatment. The situation was resolved by filing a formal complaint with police, which was successfully used to act synergistically toward the setting of appropriate therapeutic limits and the enhancement of the therapeutic relationship.

## CONCLUSIONS

Child and adolescent psychiatrists should not be intimidated by the complexities of forensic issues encountered in everyday practice. Forensic knowledge complements clinical skills. Psychiatrists must be knowledgeable about laws, regulations, and court decisions, and, at the same time, they must be open to applying creative solutions to any forensic problems encountered. In practice, the courts have purposefully delegated specific mental health decisions to expert professionals. Child and adolescent psychiatrists must take great care in and responsibility for conscientiously exercising, and not abusing, their power. If these principles are followed, children and adolescents will receive the best and fairest interventions possible in their troubled worlds.

## REFERENCES

Appelbaum, P. S., & Gutheil, T. G. (1991). *Clinical handbook of psychiatry and the law* (2d ed.). Baltimore, MD: Williams & Wilkins.

Benedek, E. P. (1992). Ethical issues in practice. In D. H. Schetky & E. P. Benedek (Eds.), *Clinical handbook of child psychiatry and the law* (pp. 75–88). Baltimore, MD: Williams & Wilkins.

Burlingame, W. V., & Amaya, M. (1992). Psychiatric commitment of children and adolescents. In D. H. Schetky & E. P. Benedek (Eds.), *Clinical handbook of child psychiatry and the law* (pp. 292–307). Baltimore, MD: Williams & Wilkins.

*In re Gault,* 387 U.S. 1 (1967).

Kalogerakis, M. G. (1992). Juvenile delinquency. In D. H. Schetky & E. P. Benedek (Eds.), *Clinical handbook of child psychiatry and the law* (pp. 191–215). Baltimore, MD: Williams & Wilkins.

Kriechman, A. M. (1989). The adolescent right to psychiatric care. In R. Rosnor & H. I. Schwartz (Eds.), *Critical issues in American psychiatry and the law: Vol. 4. Juvenile psychiatry and the law* (pp. 381–390). New York: Plenum.

Macbeth, J. E. (1992). Legal issues in the psychiatric treatment of minors. In D. H. Schetky & E. P. Benedek (Eds.), *Clinical handbook of child psychiatry and the law* (pp. 53–74). Baltimore, MD: Williams & Wilkins.

*Parham v. J.R.,* 442 U.S. 584 (1979).

Robson, K. S. (1992). Foreword. In D. H. Schetky & E. P. Benedek (Eds.), *Clinical handbook of child psychiatry and the law* (p. vii). Baltimore, MD: Williams & Wilkins.

Schetky, D. H. (1992). The child forensic evaluation. In D. H. Schetky & E. P. Benedek (Eds.), *Clinical handbook of child psychiatry and the law* (pp. 5–21). Baltimore, MD: Williams & Wilkins.

# 9

# Ethical and Forensic Considerations in Substance Abuse Treatment

HYUNG KON LEE AND
HARVEY BLUESTONE

The Epidemiological Catchment Area Study (Robins et al., 1984) carried out by the National Institute of Mental Health indicated that substance abuse disorders are the most common psychiatric problems. Drug abuse, particularly of "crack" cocaine, has been highly publicized in recent years because of its acute and severe impact on personal life, family stability, and societal welfare. However, alcohol is still the most widely abused psychoactive substance. An estimated 18 million alcoholics in the United States continue to destroy life and property to the extent that the projected cost to society was of the order of $136 billion in 1990 alone (Harwood, Kristiansen, & Rachal, 1985).

It is difficult to assess accurately the extent of alcohol's contribution to mortality. Van Natta and colleagues (Van Natta et al., 1984/1985) argue that the 3% of deaths officially attributed to alcohol in the United States represents a considerable underestimation. In addition to deaths resulting from the medical consequences of chronic alcohol use, notably, chronic liver disease and cirrhosis, alcohol has been implicated in accidental deaths involving vehicle crashes, falls, drownings, and fire. In 1987, 46,386 people died in vehicle crashes in the United States, and approximately half of these fatalities were attributable to alcohol use (National Highway Traffic Safety Administration

[NHTSA], 1988). Honkanen and co-workers (Honkanen et al., 1983) reported that 53% of 313 patients who were brought to the emergency room after accidental falls had blood alcohol concentrations (BAC) above 0.2%, which is twice the level of legal intoxication in most states. Baker, O'Neil, and Karpf (1984) found that approximately 13,000 people die as the result of alcohol-related falls every year in this country. Other studies indicate that some 48% of persons suffering fatal burns (Howland & Hingson, 1987) and 38% of those who drown (Howland & Hingson, 1988) are intoxicated at the time of their deaths. In addition, it has been reported that 20% to 36% of suicide victims used alcohol shortly before the suicidal act (Colliver & Malin, 1986; Roizen, 1982).

In a study in which all newly admitted adult inpatients were screened for alcoholism, Moore and colleagues (Moore et al., 1989) noted an overall 25% positive screening, whereas the treating physicians identified alcoholism as a problem substantially less frequently; for example, less than 10% of gynecology patients who had been screened positive were diagnosed for an alcohol problem. Yet Moore et al. found that simply telling patients their diagnosis with the suggestion that they stop drinking had a motivational effect. Physicians tend to focus on treating secondary conditions resulting from chronic alcohol consumption, but they often fail to correctly identify the patient's problems in totality. Considering the devastating consequences of alcohol abuse, and the potential benefits of early identification, the physician's failure to recognize and address the patient's alcoholism raises serious questions of ethical responsibility.

Trends such as the disease concept of addiction, the emergence of strict confidentiality provisions, and advocacy movements have raised public awareness and facilitated the process of "coming out of the closet." When alcoholism was viewed as a moral weakness and an act of willful wrongdoing, it was doubly difficult for alcoholics to come forth for treatment. The disease concept provided some relief from the burden of shame and guilt because alcoholics now could say: "It's not my fault. I have a sickness that needs to be treated." The American Medical Association (AMA) declared in 1966 that alcoholism is a disease. Subsequently, the AMA's House of Delegates adopted policies at its 1987 Annual Meeting endorsing the proposition that drug dependencies, including alcoholism, are diseases and that their treatment thus is a legitimate part of medical practice. The disease concept suffered a temporary setback in 1988 when the U.S. Supreme Court, opining that alcoholism was "willful misconduct," ruled against veterans who were seeking education benefits on the basis of alcoholism-related disability. Responding to outcries by medical and veterans groups, the U.S. Congress passed a bill, as part of the Veterans Benefits and Programs Improvement Act of 1988, in an attempt to void the Court's ruling. Despite the disease concept, the negative attitude of U.S. society toward substance abusers lingered on, and it became necessary to enact strict legislative provisions to protect the confidentiality of patients who seek treatment.

Another movement that has heightened public awareness of the need to confront alcohol abuse has been the initiative of advocacy groups such as Mothers Against Drunk Driving (MADD) and Students Against Drunk Driving (SADD). Such local movements have helped to raise the legal drinking age to 21 in many states, and have led to the legislating of stricter laws against drunk driving. Recent statistics indicate a decrease of fatal crashes involving teenage drunk drivers (NHTSA, 1988).

The nation's capacity for providing treatment to drug abusers is grossly inadequate. It is estimated that there are approximately a half million heroin addicts in the United States (Kozel & Adams, 1986). New York City, where half of the addicts live, currently has only about 35,000 slots in its methadone maintenance treatment facilities—the primary treatment modality for heroin addiction. Meanwhile, untreated abusers represent a continuing disruption of their personal and family lives, and remain both threats and burdens to society. Furthermore, the epidemic of the acquired immunodeficiency syndrome (AIDS) has increased the urgency to provide adequate treatment for drug addicts, particularly intravenous drug abusers. The New York City Department of Health's (1991) update on AIDS indicated that 46% of all AIDS cases reported in the city involved intravenous drug abusers. A recently published study by Lee, Travin, and Bluestone (1992) showed that even alcoholics and nonintravenous drug abusers had a fourfold increase in human immunodeficiency virus (HIV) seropositivity as compared with non-substance abusers among psychiatric inpatients. The presence of such a large number of HIV-seropositive patients in substance abuse treatment settings raises many ethical and legal concerns in terms of confidentiality and case management.

## CONFIDENTIALITY ISSUES IN
## SUBSTANCE ABUSE TREATMENT

Historically, alcoholics were viewed as individuals with a diminished sense of morality and limited self-discipline, and were looked down on as basically indecent or of bad character. Fears that such negative perceptions would lead to discrimination or outright rejection were clearly a potential obstacle to alcoholics who would otherwise seek treatment. To protect individuals' privacy, and to eliminate such unnecessary fears or concerns, current federal law provides protection against unauthorized disclosure of information related to alcohol and drug treatment.

A Department of Health and Human Services (1987) regulation prohibits disclosure or use of such patient records except in certain specific circumstances. To disclose information, the patient must consent in writing, and the disclosed information must be accompanied by a statement that prohibits further disclosure. The regulations permit disclosure without patient consent if the disclosure is to medical personnel to meet a bona fide medical emergency. It also permits disclosure to qualified personnel for research, audit, or program evaluation, but the qualified personnel may not include patient-identifying information in any report or otherwise disclose patient identity. The regulations permit disclosure pursuant to a court order after the court has made a finding that "good cause" exists. Each patient must be told about these confidentiality provisions and must be furnished a summary in writing.

For methadone maintenance treatment patients, confidentiality issues are more complex, involving not only drug treatment confidentiality, but also strict provisions concerning disclosure of HIV status.

### Case 1: Confidentiality Issues for an HIV-Positive
### Methadone Maintenance Patient

Ms. A., a 34-year-old, single woman with a 14-year history of heroin abuse, has been a patient of a methadone maintenance treatment program for two years. She lives in her own apartment with her boyfriend and her two children, aged four and six. She is unemployed and receives public assistance. Since her admission to the methadone maintenance treatment program, she has abstained from heroin use, but her drinking has escalated to a daily consumption of 10–12 cans of beer. She also has begun to smoke crack at a cost of $80 to $100 daily. Occasionally, Ms. A. has come to the clinic accompanied by her two small children, who appeared poorly groomed and malnourished. Although she insists that she is a good mother and has had no difficulty in taking care of the children, there is a strong suspicion that the children are neglected.

In view of Ms. A.'s complaints of fatigue, weight loss, coughing, and low-grade fever, coupled with her long history of intravenous drug abuse, she was advised to have an HIV test. She consented in writing after receiving pretest counseling, which included an explanation of the nature of HIV infection and related illness and the benefits of taking the test, information regarding discrimination problems and confidentiality provisions, and information on preventing the transmission of HIV. Upon testing positive, she was provided with posttest counseling that addressed ways of coping emotionally with the test result, discrimination issues, confidentiality issues, prevention of HIV transmission, availability of medical treatment, and the need to notify contacts. Ms. A. rejected the advice to inform her boyfriend of her HIV status, and she specifically instructed the clinic staff not to inform him. She also admitted that they were not practicing safe sex. Ms. A. asked her social worker to write a letter to the Department of Social Services stating that she was attending the program, but said that she did not want to disclose her HIV status to anybody.

The clinic staff took the following actions: (1) After obtaining written consent from the patient, a letter was sent to the Department of Social Services stating that she was attending the program as scheduled. (2) The clinic physician referred her to a medical clinic for evaluation, and her HIV status was noted in the referral letter. (3) The clinic staff expressed concern about the possible neglect of the children and offered her a home visit. When she refused the offer, the clinic social worker alerted the child abuse protective agency. (4) The clinic physician felt that Ms. A.'s boyfriend needed to be protected from transmission of HIV and should have a medical evaluation, and he contacted the man without identifying the patient or the clinic. The boyfriend was advised to receive HIV counseling because he had been exposed to the virus.

*Discussion of Case 1*

This case presents several ethical and legal issues that clinicians frequently encounter in treating substance abusers. Many substance abusers are referred to treatment programs by social service agencies, which have an interest in preventing beneficiaries from using public assistance funds to procure alcohol or drugs. Despite their reluctance to enter treatment, addicted individuals feel compelled to enroll in the treatment program in order to secure such income. Whatever the motives may be, it is a positive change for these individuals to have an opportunity to participate in treatment processes. However, often the primary objective is to maintain public assistance benefits, rather than to accomplish treatment goals by attending the program on a regular basis. While clinicians owe a duty of loyalty to their patients, they also have ethical responsibilities to society. Thus clinicians must carefully assess the degree of meaningful participation by patients before writing letters certifying their participation status. Routinely furnishing a preprinted letter, regardless of the degree of a patient's participation, that indicates that the patient is enrolled in the program may be misleading and ethically wrong.

Considering the devastating consequences of HIV transmission, some states, such as New York, permit a physician to notify partner(s) of an HIV-positive individual without the patient's consent, although the patient remains anonymous. However, the law does not require such notification. Thus physicians are left in the uncomfortable position of having to decide whether to notify. The American Psychiatric Association's (APA) code of ethics is equally vague by stating that a physician may notify partners. The rationale for informing partners without identifying the patient is to protect the confidentiality and privacy of the infected person.

In Ms. A.'s case, it would not be difficult for her boyfriend to figure out that the individual whom the physician did not want to identify was his girlfriend. Additionally, the patient will eventually learn that her doctor was the one who informed him. Hence the merit of anonymous notification is dubious, and it may further erode trust between physician and patient. Physicians may have an ethical obligation to inform partners of HIV-positive individuals of possible exposure to the virus, but it may be therapeutically advisable to discuss the intent to notify in advance with the patient.

Although it is important to maintain strict confidentiality in substance abuse treatment, the government has recognized an even more urgent need to protect children from neglect or abuse by substance abusers, who are particularly prone to engage in such behavior (Bland & Orn, 1986). The federal confidentiality law stipulates that, if an alcohol- or drug-abuse-service provider suspects child abuse or neglect by a patient, and desires to comply with state reporting requirements, the provider can enter into a "qualified service organization agreement" with the appropriate child abuse protective agency. Under the agreement, the child abuse protective agency is bound by the confidentiality regulations with respect to patient information obtained from the service provider. This provision permits the child abuse protective statute effectively to override the confidentiality law of alcohol or drug abuse treatment records.

Notably, clinicians do not require proof of abuse or neglect in order to make a report. Reporting does not indicate that abuse or neglect actually occurred, but rather that there is cause for investigation. It is disputable as to at what point the clinician needs to report potential child abuse or neglect. Some clinicians contend that alcohol or drug abuse by a mother of young children is sufficient reason to report. While this approach may be disputable, clinicians have an unquestionable legal and ethical responsibility to alert the child abuse protective agency when there is a strong suspicion of child abuse or neglect, as illustrated in Ms. A.'s case.

## TREATMENT BY COERCION

In principle, substance abuse treatment is initiated and carried out on a voluntary basis. However, there are instances in which individuals are compelled to enroll in substance abuse treatment. A case in point is driving while intoxicated (DWI) treatment programs. The majority of patients enrolled in DWI treatment programs do not believe that they need treatment, yet they see no other choice but to participate in order to satisfy judicial requirements. New York State law stipulates a $350 fine and/or one-year imprisonment, in addition to a six-month license revocation, for the first DWI offense, and a $500 fine and/or four years' imprisonment, in addition to a one-year license revocation, for the second DWI offense.

In many instances, however, education and treatment are preferable to punitive measures. Thus, in 1975, New York State established its Alcohol and Drug Rehabilitation Program, commonly known as the Drinking Driver Program (DDP). The goal of DDP is to educate social drinkers, and to refer for treatment those with serious alcohol or drug problems. Often the referrals are made to DWI treatment programs. While any drunk driving offender can be admitted to an educational program, the clinician must establish evidence that the individual suffers from a diagnosable medical condition, either alcohol abuse or dependence, in order to admit the person to a DWI treatment program. This technical issue at times creates difficulties in making admission decisions.

To make a diagnosis of alcohol abuse disorder, the APA *Diagnostic and Statistical Manual of Mental Disorders,* revised third edition (DSM-III-R) (1987), requires a maladaptive pattern of alcohol use indicated by (1) continued use despite knowledge of having a persistent or recurrent social, occupational, psychological, or physical problem that is caused or exacerbated by use of alcohol, or (2) recurrent use in situations in which the use is physically hazardous. Individuals referred to DWI treatment programs, and even their significant others, frequently blame "bad luck" for their predicament and deny having any alcohol-related problem. In these circumstances, the only criterion that can positively establish the diagnosis of alcohol abuse is "recurrent" use in situations in which the use is physically hazardous. If an individual has been convicted for drunk driving more than once, the alcohol-abuse diagnosis is not controversial. However, if a person is referred to a DWI treatment program for the first offense, and he or she denies alcohol consumption since the drunk driving arrest, assignment of an alcohol-abuse diagnosis becomes a more controversial task.

Upon admission to the treatment program, DWI patients have little option but to comply with recommended treatment as long as they wish to maintain or regain possession of a driver's license. Thus the program effectively can utilize a wide range of treatment options with increased compliance. A case in point is Antabuse (disulfiram) treatment. At the Bronx-Lebanon Hospital, DWI program patients who fail to maintain sobriety are offered alternative treatment modalities, such as Antabuse treatment or inpatient detoxification and rehabilitation. In a majority of cases, patients choose to take Antabuse, and the program requires them to take the medication under the supervision of a staff member because such an approach has been found to be effective (Sereny et al., 1986). One may question whether such a coercive approach is ethically correct. However, ethical correctness must be considered in the context of serving the patient and safeguarding the public.

## Case 2: Treatment in a DWI Program

Mr. B. is a 37-year-old married man with four children. He works as a driver for a limousine company. Mr. B. stated that he started to drink at age 21, and that he is a social drinker who occasionally drinks one or two cans of beer with friends. He denied any unusual behavior when he drinks, but said that he "can express himself better." He also denied any history of blackouts, morning shakes, hallucinations, or seizures. Mr. B. asserted that he was trying to move his car to the opposite side of the street after drinking two cans of beer when he was arrested. He maintained that he did not have any previous drunk driving arrests or any other legal problem. He complained that the arresting officer was unfair because he was not going to drive anywhere, but was just trying to move his car across the street. He refused to take a breath analyzer test because he was angry at the officer. Mr. B. pled guilty to a lesser charge of "driving while his ability was impaired" (BAC 0.05–0.09%) instead of driving while intoxicated (BAC 0.1% or greater) in order to avoid "wasting time" by going back and forth to court. He was granted a conditional license with the stipulation that he participate in a drunk driver education program. In the sixth week of the program, alcohol was detected on his breath and he was referred to a DWI treatment program.

When Mr. B. was examined by a physician at the DWI treatment program, he angrily denounced the decision to send him for treatment after "wasting" six weeks at the education program. He said that he was continuing to drink "socially" because he did not think he was a problem drinker, and that he would not drive when he drank. On examination, Mr. B. was found to be an angry and impulsive person, and it was difficult to elicit a reliable drinking history because of his pervasive denial and rationalization. Otherwise, his mental-status examination was unremarkable. After obtaining Mr. B.'s permission, his wife was invited for an interview for further diagnostic clarification. She was protective of her husband and denied that he had any problem with drinking. However, she acknowledged that her husband suffered from a peptic ulcer. The physician decided to recommend treatment in the DWI treatment program on the basis of (1) conviction for drunk driving, (2) continued drinking despite the arrest, and (3) continued drinking while suffering from an ulcer. Mr. B. strongly protested the doctor's decision, and he was advised that he could obtain a second opinion. When a second physician made the same recommendation, Mr. B. decided to appeal his conviction. However, he later returned to the DWI program for treatment because his lawyer had advised him against the appeal.

*Discussion of Case 2*

The case described illustrates a dilemma that a DWI program physician may face from time to time. The physician understood that this was not a "clear-cut case" and his decision to recommend treatment had to be made on assumptions. Although Mr. B. could be correct in saying that he did not need to stop drinking because he was a "social drinker," the physician had to believe that he had consumed a substantial quantity of alcohol at the time of his arrest because conviction for drunk driving requires collateral evidence of intoxication, in addition to the refusal of a breath analyzer test. Additionally, the fact that he drove to the education program with a detectable odor of alcohol on his breath contradicted his claim that he would not drive when he drank. Finally, the physician had to assess carefully the potential consequences of admitting or not admitting him to the program. An erroneous decision to admit him might cause financial loss or emotional pain to Mr. B. and his family. On the other hand, an erroneous decision not to admit him might result in serious consequences to the public. In the final analysis, the physician made the decision he believed most prudent and recommended treatment. This recommendation essentially mandated treatment because failure to comply with the recommendation in effect constitutes failure to satisfy judicial requirements. The physician, at the same time, did not pretend that his decision was absolute, and allowed the client to obtain a second opinion. This approach was an attempt to develop a positive therapeutic relationship between the physician and patient.

## IMPAIRED PHYSICIAN

In 1973, the AMA's Council on Mental Health issued a report on "The Sick Physician," which defined physician impairment as the inability to practice medicine adequately by reason of physical or mental illness, including alcoholism or drug dependence. Since then, most state medical societies have formed impaired-physicians committees. Although the approaches of these committees vary from state to state, several societies place primary emphasis on alcoholism and/or drug abuse.

It is speculated that a physician's access to controlled drugs may increase the risk of abuse of such drugs. In addition, occupation-related stresses may present vulnerability to a variety of physical and emotional disorders, as well as to alcohol or drug abuse (Pearson, 1982). Vaillant's (Vaillant, Sobowale, & McArthur, 1975) study of 46 physicians over a 30-year period revealed that 36% of them developed alcohol and/or drug (including tranquilizer) abuse as compared with 22% among nonphysician controls. Other studies (Dorr, 1982; Hill, Haertzen, & Yamahiro, 1968) show that addicted physicians may reveal long-standing personality traits, such as defensive, obsessive-compulsive, and depressive characteristics. The life of the impaired physician becomes progressively more chaotic and erratic. Eventually, changes in his or her behavior and medical practice will become unmistakable, and yet, traditionally, physicians have been highly reluctant to confront and remedy such problems. However, increasing public criticism of the medical profession's inability to protect the public from harm caused by impaired or incompetent physicians has led to the enactment of impaired-physician statutes in many states. Similarly, the medical profession has responded by creating impaired-physicians committees to identify and assist their impaired members. While some societies act as the state disciplinary body, others are required to report a physician's misconduct to the state disciplinary agency. In New York State, individual practitioners are required by statute to report physician misconduct to a state disciplinary body. Furthermore, failure to report can itself constitute misconduct.

### Case 3: Impaired Physician

Dr. C., a 45-year-old surgeon, was referred by the county medical society to a psychiatrist who acted as a consultant to the society's impaired-physicians committee. Dr. C. had a 25-year history of drinking. He explained that he used to drink only a few cans of beer at week-end social functions until he went through a bitter divorce battle five years previously. His drinking escalated to a pint of liquor daily "just to forget problems." About a year earlier, he had started to experience hand tremors upon awakening in the morning. To control the withdrawal symptoms, he used samples of benzodiazepine tranquilizers, at times supplemented by prescriptions he wrote himself.

Dr. C.'s colleagues had suspected that something was wrong with him because of the steady deterioration of his personal grooming and his frequent absences. Finally, one day, while he was operating on a patient, his assistant observed that Dr. C.'s hands were getting increasingly shaky and unsteady. The assistant completed the procedure and then reported the incident to the chief of service, who in turn reported it to the appropriate state investigating agency. When Dr. C. realized the serious nature of his predicament, he asked the county medical society for assistance. The medical society in turn requested a psychiatric evaluation. On examination, Dr. C. minimized his problem by saying that he had drunk a little too much the night before the surgery, but that he really did not think that he had a drinking problem. He felt that everything would be all right if he took a vacation. After further interviews and confrontations, he reluctantly agreed to enter an alcoholism rehabilitation program. The consultant recommended a program specially designed for addicted health-care professionals. Additionally, the consultant advised Dr. C. not to return to medical practice until a satisfactory rehabilitation was accomplished, and Dr. C. agreed.

*Discussion of Case 3*

Although the substance-abusing physician may make every effort to preserve his or her ability to function professionally, changes in behavior and professional performance may become obvious. But even when such changes become evident, colleagues may deny the seriousness of the problem (Shapiro, 1975) or look the other way because they feel that reporting the impaired physician may be seen as an act of betrayal and contribute to a suffering colleague's difficulties. It appears that Dr. C.'s colleagues were no exception. They either denied or avoided the problem until it became obvious that Dr. C.'s patient was in jeopardy. However, once it reached that critical point, his colleagues and the hospital authorities took action to correct the situation by reporting it and advising him to seek help. Dr. C. wisely decided to find help voluntarily. The state disciplinary agency agreed to take no action on his license status provided that he undergo alcohol rehabilitation treatment and submit progress reports at regular intervals. Although the hospital authorities satisfied their legal obligation by reporting Dr. C.'s case to the state investigating agency, the hospital's responsibility for safeguarding patients still had to be addressed in terms of making a decision on Dr. C.'s hospital privileges.

Galanter and colleagues (Galanter et al., 1990) studied 100 physicians who had completed Georgia's Impaired Physicians Program, which included four weeks in the hospital, 15 weeks in a transitional residence, and aftercare groups with an Alcoholics Anonymous (AA)-like format. An average 33.4 months after admission to the program, only 14 indicated that they had used alcohol or drugs since entering the program. None reported drug abuse within the past month. All but five were practicing medicine. Unquestionably, there is an overwhelming incentive for physicians to succeed in such treatment. Whatever the contributing factors might be, these positive findings amply justify a licensing board's efforts to compel an impaired physician to accept a rehabilitation program rather than to resort to punitive action. Physicians must realize that identifying and reporting impaired colleagues who are in desperate need of help is not betraying or hurting the suffering colleague. On the contrary, such action can offer impaired colleagues an opportunity to rehabilitate their lives and, with their knowledge and skills, continue contributing to society.

## REFERENCES

American Medical Association, Council on Mental Health. (1973). The sick physician. *JAMA, 223,* 684–687.

American Psychiatric Association. (1987). *Diagnostic and statistical manual of mental disorders* (3d ed., rev.). Washington, DC: American Psychiatric Press.

Baker, S. P., O'Neil, B., & Karpf, R. (1984). *Injury fact book.* Lexington, MA: Heath.

Bland, R., & Orn, H. (1986). Family violence and psychiatric disorder. *Canadian Journal of Psychiatry, 31,* 129–137.

Colliver, J. D., & Malin, H. (1986). State and national trends in alcohol related mortality: 1975–1982. *Alcohol Health and Research World, 10,* 60–64, 75.

Department of Health and Human Services, Public Health Service. (1987). 42 CFR Part II: Confidentiality of alcohol and drug abuse patient records. *Federal Register,* June 9.

Dorr, D. (1982). MMPI profile of emotionally impaired physicians. *Psychiatric Annals, 12,* 238–244.

Galanter, M., Talbott, D., Gallegos, K., et al. (1990). Combined alcoholics anonymous and professional care for addicted physicians. *American Journal of Psychiatry, 147,* 64–68.

Harwood, H. J., Kristiansen, P., & Rachal, J. V. (1985). Social and economic costs of alcohol abuse and alcoholism. *Issue report no. 2.* Research Triangle Park, NC: Research Triangle Institute.

Hill, H. E., Haertzen, C. A., & Yamahiro, R. S. (1968). The addict physician: A Minnesota Multiphasic Personality Inventory study of the interaction of personality characteristics and availability of narcotics. In A. Wickler (Ed.), *The addictive states.* Baltimore, MD: Williams & Wilkins.

Honkanen, R., Ertama, L., Kuosmanen, P., et al. (1983). The role of alcohol in accidental falls. *Journal of Studies in Alcohol, 44,* 231–245.

Howland, J., & Hingson, R. (1987). Alcohol as risk factor for injuries or deaths due to fires and burns: Review of literature. *Public Health Report, 102,* 475–483.

Howland, J., & Hingson, R. (1988). Issues in research on alcohol in nonvehicular unintentional injuries. *Contemporary Drug Problems*, Spring, 95–106.

Kozel, N. J., & Adams, E. H. (1986). Epidemiology of drug abuse: An overview. *Science, 234*, 970–974.

Lee, H. K., Travin, S., & Bluestone, H. (1992). Relationship between HIV-1 antibody seropositivity and alcohol/nonintravenous drug abuse among psychiatric inpatients. *American Journal of Addictions, 1*, 85–88.

Moore, R. D., Bone, L. R., Geller, G., et al. (1989). Prevalence, detection and treatment of alcoholism in hospitalized patients. *JAMA, 261*, 403–407.

National Highway Traffic Safety Administration (NHTSA), National Center for Statistics and Analysis. (1988). *Drunk driving facts*. Washington, DC: Author.

New York City Department of Health. (1991). *AIDS surveillance update*. New York.

Pearson, M. M. (1982). Psychiatric treatment of 250 physicians. *Psychiatric Annals, 12*, 194–206.

Robins, L. E., Helzer, J. E., Weissman, M. M., et al. (1984). Lifetime prevalence of specific psychiatric disorders in three sites. *Archives of General Psychiatry, 41*, 949–958.

Roizen, J. (1982). Estimating alcohol involvement in serious events. In National Institute on Alcohol Abuse and Alcoholism, *Alcohol consumption and related problems* (Alcohol and Health Monograph No. 1) (DHHS Pub. No. [ADM] 82-1190) (pp. 179–219). Washington, DC: U.S. Government Printing Office.

Sereny, G., Sharma, V., Holt, J., et al. (1986). Mandatory supervised Antabuse therapy in an outpatient alcoholism program: A pilot study. *Alcoholism, 10*, 290–296.

Shapiro, E. T. (1975). The mentally ill physician as practitioner. *JAMA, 232*, 725–727.

Vaillant, G. E., Sobowale, N. C., & McArthur, C. (1975). Some psychologic vulnerabilities of physicians. *New England Journal of Medicine, 287*, 372–375.

Van Natta, P., Malin, H., Bertolucci, D., et al. (1984/1985). The hidden influence of alcohol on mortality (Epidemiologic Bulletin No. 6). *Alcohol Health and Research World, 9*, 42–45.

# 10

# Partial Hospitalization and Intensive Outpatient Management in the General Hospital
## A Unique Clinicolegal Status

DOUGLAS B. MARLOWE,
ALLAN M. TEPPER, AND
ELISABETH N. GIBBINGS

Partial hospitalization and intensive outpatient management are generally considered effective and cost-efficient alternatives to inpatient psychiatric treatment. While designed to provide many of the services available in an inpatient setting, these programs seek to avoid the regressive and disruptive influences of institutionalization by maintaining community ties; enhancing adaptive functioning (daily living skills, social competence, work, education); and avoiding stigmatizing labels (e.g., Hoge, Farrell, Strauss, & Posner, 1987; Schreer, 1988). Available studies suggest that, in the long term, such intensive, longitudinal care is more efficient than intermittent inpatient hospitalization,

Substantial portions of this paper appeared in *Comprehensive Mental Health Care* (Marlowe, Tepper, & Gibbings, 1992).

Unless otherwise indicated, the term "partial program" is used generically to refer to partial or day hospitals proper, as well as intensive outpatient programs, that employ various group therapies and skills training in a stable therapeutic milieu.

reducing the debilitating and costly effects of "revolving door" admissions (e.g., Cuyler, 1991; Weiss & Dubin, 1982).

Although originally conceived as a form of community-based treatment, partial programs have actually migrated toward and flourished in general and free-standing psychiatric hospitals (Weiss & Dubin, 1982). The deinstitutionalization movement of the 1960s witnessed the demise of vast state psychiatric institutions and the proliferation of novel treatment models. However, the movement ultimately failed in its stated goal of creating a community-based treatment and support network (Mental Retardation and Community Health Centers Construction Act, 1963) to absorb the newly released institutionalized populations (Bach, 1989). As a result, the general hospital was relegated the responsibility of providing health care for a new class of disenfranchised, chronic psychiatric patients, necessitating a precipitous expansion of alternative treatment programs.

Notably, because this proliferation resulted from a sudden confluence of social, political, and economic forces, there has been little opportunity for the appropriate evolution and evaluation of these programs. As Cuyler (1991) recently concluded, "[M]arketplace forces have a way of promoting much more rapid change in the delivery of health care than do advances in clinical knowledge. The decade ahead may very well see growing acceptance of partial hospitalization and rapid development of new programs—perhaps without an opportunity for gradual, planned maturity" (p. 48). In fact, the field is at such an early stage of development that these programs are only broadly defined. Officially, partial hospitalization is vaguely conceived as "a time-limited, ambulatory, active treatment program that offers therapeutically intensive, coordinated, and structured clinical services within a stable therapeutic milieu" (American Association for Partial Hospitalization [AAPH], 1991a, p. 1; see also National Association of Private Psychiatric Hospitals [NAPPH] & AAPH, 1990).

Similarly, legal and professional regulation has lagged behind program development, giving little guidance to mental health professionals who seek to implement and promote these programs in an ethically defensible manner. To date, there is only a limited number of regulatory bodies that have begun promulgating standards and guidelines for partial programs (see AAPH, 1991a, 1991b; NAPPH & AAPH,

1990; Joint Commission on Accreditation of Healthcare Organizations [JCAHO], 1991). These regulations focus almost exclusively on clinical and administrative—as opposed to legal—considerations. It should be noted, however, that in the absence of an adequate body of legal authority, courts may take judicial notice of industry standards, giving them the practical effect of law (*Darling v. Charleston Community Memorial Hospital,* 1965). Yet adherence to such guidelines does not ensure protection from liability, as courts feel free to reject the standards of an "infant" profession if the evolution of its ethical guidelines is deemed insufficient or "unreasonable" (*Helling v. Carey,* 1974).

In the absence of clear legal precedent, clinicians rightfully feel vulnerable to malpractice or tort liability, and they fear loss of program accreditation (and thus access to elusive third-party reimbursement [Weiss & Dubin, 1982]). How can professionals working in general hospital partial programs protect themselves from liability? Generally speaking, the answer is to equate clinical and legal requirements. As noted, the courts will incorporate reasonable clinical practice into the legal standard of care.

Of course, the difficulty is in applying this broad principle in daily practice. In the absence of clear authority, we recommend the following "litmus test." In evaluating a potential course of action, the clinician should ask himself or herself: (1) Would I feel comfortable defending this action before a group of my colleagues? (2) Can I ground the rationale for the action in explicit professional ethical principles, institutional bylaws, quality assurance mandates, and so on? (3) If the action differs from what I would do in a purely inpatient or outpatient setting, can I justify this deviation in terms of differences in practice context? and, (4) If the action differs from what I have done before, what makes this situation different (e.g., more regressed patient, different physical plant, smaller staff)? If unable to answer these questions comfortably, the clinician should reconsider the intended course of action.

Of course, in many instances, reasonable professionals could reach different conclusions about the appropriate course of action. Further, it is not unusual to rationalize an ill-chosen decision after the fact. That is why legal and ethical precedent evolves gradually in a case-by-case manner. Yet a number of recurrent issues facing clinicians in hospital-based partial programs have surfaced. In the remainder of this chapter, we present some of these commonly confronted dilemmas and implement an explicit ethical decision-making process.

## CONSTRUCTION OF THE MILIEU

Dr. Tuferwun was recently appointed director of outpatient services in the psychiatric department of a general hospital. She was given a mandate from the administration to develop a financially profitable partial program, which would also alleviate the census burden on the general outpatient clinic and serve as a primary aftercare resource for the psychiatry, neurology and medical/surgical units.

To contain start-up costs, Dr. Tuferwun decided that all partial-hospital patients would join the psychiatric inpatient milieu and follow the same morning schedule (group therapy, community meeting, creative arts therapy, and lunch). This arrangement would lower physical plant utilization by 8%, and would require a 15% lower staff-to-patient ratio. Dr. Tuferwun also reasoned that the partial-hospital patients would benefit from treatment by the experienced inpatient staff, and the adaptive skills of the inpatients would improve through exposure to their higher functioning peers.

### Location of the Program

It is common practice for hospital-based partial programs to be integrated in some manner into existing inpatient services (Javorsky, 1992). Obviously, duplication of plant and program usage lowers operational costs. Further, from a clinical standpoint, patients might benefit from interaction with peers at divergent levels of functioning and stages of recovery. For example, contact with lower functioning individuals may help put one's situation in perspective, while interaction with less regressed patients may raise the psychosocial level of the milieu (Hoge & McLoughlin, 1991; Weiss & Dubin, 1982). Higher functioning patients can serve as role models for more regressed patients, while being reminded of their own treatment gains (or absence thereof).

However, a number of clinical and administrative (and thus legal and ethical) factors may dictate separate treatment for partial-program patients. When in acute crisis, patients require a contained (and perhaps locked) space in order to regulate extraneous traffic and stimulation. Isolation from excessive sights and sounds is itself therapeutic. Generally speaking, however, partial-program patients are in a less regressed state than inpatients. Presumably they have a higher stimulus threshold and more intact personal (ego) boundaries (Cuyler, 1991; Kennedy, 1991; Klar, Frances, & Clarkin, 1982). In contrast to inpatients, they require stimulation to improve their interest in, and engagement with, the environment, and confinement could thus be countertherapeutic.

Although, as noted, there are potential benefits to mixing different classes of patients in groups or treatment programs, there is also a concomitant risk of "group casualty" (Galinsky & Schopler, 1977, p. 89; Parker, 1976). In particular, patients manifesting such "vulnerability factors" (Keith-Spiegel & Koocher, 1985, p. 137) as impaired reality testing, diffuse ego boundaries, intense fear of rejection, excessive dependency, and social withdrawal may be at risk for serious decompensation if they fall short of excessive group expectations, becoming ostracized by or prey to manipulative and more integrated members. Program directors must always be sensitive to each participant's appropriateness for the milieu, regardless of the setting. The legal and ethical implications of this issue are highlighted when different classes of patients (partial, outpatient, or inpatient) are combined for apparently economic motives.

There is also the potential that the partial-hospital patients' treatment will be negatively affected by integration with a more regressed population. It is certainly not unusual for psychiatric inpatients to have a dampening effect on group process. Further, as it is necessary for group therapists to treat groups at a psychosocial level commensurate with the "lowest common denominator," there is a likelihood that higher functioning patients will be insufficiently engaged and their needs ignored. Thus, if the tone of an inpatient milieu is disorganized, and the patient population is poorly related, there is less clinical and ethical justification for combining populations.

If patients and staff are given the covert message that partial treatment is no different than traditional inpatient care, the nature and level of the partial care will undoubtedly "degrade" accordingly (Bendit, 1991). In the above vignette, it is unlikely that Dr. Tuferwun's staff will be able adequately to differentiate inpatients from partial-program patients and provide the corresponding structure and support. In the absence of appropriate programmatic safeguards, substandard care could be provided, leading to malpractice exposure and a potential loss of program accreditation.

## Specialized Programming and Treatment Planning

As the previous discussion illustrates, there are no bright-line rules concerning the location of partial programs. Depending on the specific context, there may be clinical justification for mixing or segregating different classes of patients. As discussed earlier, a good rule-of-thumb is for mental health professionals to ground such decisions in explicit industry and institutional standards.

The official industry formulation of partial hospitalization requires that the program furnish a "*distinct and organized* intensive ambulatory treatment service" (NAPPH & AAPH, 1990, p. 89) and that it be conceived and implemented as a "*separate, identifiable, organized unit*" (AAPH, 1991a, p. 2) (emphases added). Admittedly, such terms as "distinct," "separate," and "organized" are so vague as to be practically unenforceable. However, in common usage, these terms refer to a reasonable degree of differentiation and specialization, and it is likely that the courts would give them such a construction in determining the applicable standard of care.

The existence of partial programs is justified by the presumed specialized needs of a subset of psychiatric patients. Thus these programs must be sufficiently specialized to meet those identified needs. The closer a partial program's goals and treatment plans are to those of traditional inpatient or outpatient care, the less rationale there is for the program. Notably, such specialized programming can be accomplished regardless of whether the program is housed on an inpatient unit or in a separate building. The crucial issue is whether treatment planning and programming are conducted in a rational and specialized manner.

The official industry standard for partial hospitalization requires that an individualized, written treatment plan, documenting the patient's appropriateness for partial care, be developed by a qualified mental health professional upon initial contact with the patient (AAPH, 1991a,b; NAPPH & AAPH, 1990). As a condition of accreditation, JCAHO (1991) requires partial hospitalization programs to formulate and specify explicit methods and standards for intake, assessment, and treatment and discharge planning (including periodic review) (sec. II [1.1.1–1.1.5]). Treatment planning must be specific to the particular program, as well as to the specific needs of each patient (1.1.3). Notably, when a program deals with more regressed patients who require specialized services (e.g., Baker & McColley, 1982 [schizophrenics]; Kennedy, 1991 [borderlines]; Topp, 1991 [young children]; Wagner, 1991 [geriatrics]), there is an increased clinical and legal requirement to develop stratified treatment protocols, and to document the individual's need for treatment in a partial setting (AAPH, 1991b; Kiser, Heston, Millsap, & Pruitt, 1991).

Yet, despite industry requirements, the available evidence suggests that many partial and intensive outpatient treatment staffs do not formulate or implement adequate treatment plans, even with specialized populations (Kiser et al., 1991). For example, based on site visits to 18 child and adolescent day programs, Doan and Petti (1990) found that over one half of the treatment plans lacked mandatory periodic review. Further, justification for admission and diagnosis was "poor" on over 40% of the charts, and there was no documentation of ongoing therapist–patient contact in 44% of the cases.

Treatment planning refers to the needs of individual patients. In addition, partial programs must have specialized scheduling and programming to serve the general requirements of the particular patient population (AAPH, 1991a,b). At a minimum, the activity schedule should reflect the fundamental difference between partial and inpatient care. Partial-care patients spend most of their day away from the program, in an unregulated and stressful community environment. It is, therefore, essential for staff members to address outside issues directly, and to help patients develop generalizable problem-solving strategies.

In the above vignette, the program schedule does not satisfy even the rudiments of differentiation. For example, although there may be justification for having partial-program patients attend some inpatient activities, there is little rationale for having them join the community meeting, which presumably addresses issues related to inpatient life. Rather, it is good clinical practice to make regular morning "check-in" and afternoon "wrap-up" groups an integral part of the partial-program schedule (Bendit, 1991). Such groups explicitly recognize and capitalize on the patients' community contacts, using those experiences as "grist for the mill" to identify maladaptive behaviors and to practice alternative strategies. In the morning, patients should review their activities since the last contact and evaluate how well they have met previously set goals. If appropriate, their dress and grooming should be assessed, and they can be checked for contraband. In the afternoon group, patients should evaluate their progress for the day, set goals for the hours until the next meeting, and anticipate upcoming problems and stressors. By establishing an explicit continuity between patients' community and hospital experiences, the partial program should ultimately render itself obsolete to the needs of the particular patients.

**Appropriate Patients**

Another significant difficulty with Dr. Tuferwun's program is her failure to develop explicit criteria for determining patients' suitability for partial hospitalization. At a minimum, there must be recognition of the contraindications to any form of outpatient case management. Individuals who are grossly disorganized, or at significant risk for injury to self or others, are clearly not appropriate (AAPH, 1991a,b). Specifically, suicidal patients who do not have a secure therapeutic alliance or adequate community supports, individuals with seriously impaired self-care (activities of daily living, ADL) skills, and those manifesting behavioral disinhibition or aggression dysregulation, should not be treated in such a setting (Cuyler, 1991; Klar et al., 1982).

Another major issue is whether partial programs should include chronic or rehabilitation patients (Klar et al., 1982; Weiss & Dubin,

1982). Notably, the contemporary formulation of partial hospitalization requires that there be a "reasonable expectation for improvement," and that such treatment be "necessary to maintain [the] patient's functional level and prevent relapse or full hospitalization" (NAPPH & AAPH, 1990, p. 1). There must be a reasonable expectation that partial treatment will forestall further decompensation, which would necessitate inpatient care. Further, there must be some demonstration that less restrictive and costly treatment, such as general outpatient management, is unsuitable; that is, that the patient has failed to make gains in traditional outpatient treatment, or that the presenting complaint is so severe that success with such treatment is "doubtful" (AAPH, 1991a, p. 4; see also AAPH, 1991b; NAPPH & AAPH, 1990). In essence, if a program does not satisfy these criteria, it should not be labeled as a "partial hospital." Rather, it should be labeled a "residential" or "rehabilitation" facility or "outpatient clinic," thus triggering entirely disparate reimbursement schedules and regulatory schemes.

In the above vignette, Dr. Tuferwun should not have accepted the administration's blanket mandate to receive referrals from the neurology and medical/surgical units, as there is a high likelihood that such patients will have chronic illnesses that require rehabilitation, as opposed to acute illnesses that are amenable to active treatment or stabilization. Further, partial hospitals are conceived solely as treatment programs for psychiatric patients manifesting disorders consistent with the *Diagnostic and Statistical Manual of Mental Disorders,* revised third edition (DSM-III-R) (American Psychiatric Association, 1987) nomenclature (AAPH, 1991a,b; NAPPH & AAPH, 1990). They are inappropriate for general medical or surgical follow-up care.

To this point, we have reviewed the minimum selection criteria that must be employed. However, there are numerous other factors that should be considered in constituting a patient milieu. In broad terms, program leaders are required to "promote and maintain a stable, consistent, and cohesive therapeutic milieu or therapeutic community" (AAPH, 1991a, p. 6). Thus it is incumbent on staff members to screen, match, and orient participants in advance to promote a workable group dynamic (Keith-Spiegel & Koocher, 1985; Lakin, 1988; Rosenthal, 1987). For example, there is much controversy as to whether patients should be grouped by symptom (e.g., codependency, substance abuse), syndrome (e.g., schizophrenia, character pathology), or demographics (e.g., age, sex, race). In general, the answer should depend on the philosophy, experience, and resources of the particular program and staff. However, to ensure a workable group process, patients at least should be matched on such clinically relevant variables as general intelligence, psychosocial development, emotional vulnerability, communication (verbal or nonverbal) ability, and tolerance for interaction.

## Discharge Criteria

In addition to establishing admission criteria for partial programs, it is essential to develop standards and mechanisms for discharge and transfer. There is growing evidence that a new population of long-term-stay partial hospital patients is developing; a process described as the "new route to institutionalization" (Tantam & McGrath, 1989). Just as the past accumulation of patients on long term inpatient units undermined initiative and independence, so too may lengthy day treatment contribute to "secondary handicaps." Further, in the age of health care reform and increased accountability, it is incumbent on health care professionals to explicitly justify continued treatment; that is, to demonstrate the likelihood of meaningful or substantial improvement from partial program care, as well as the "marginal utility" of partial treatment over less costly modalities.

This requires partial program staff to formulate treatment plans with clearly articulated, measurable, and obtainable goals. An identifiable endpoint of partial treatment should be anticipated. Ideally, the minutes from treatment team meetings, as well as individual patient charts, should make explicit reference to these goals, documenting patients' gains or apparent reasons for the absence of gains. A good practice in team meetings is for staff members from various disciplines (e.g., the primary therapist, social worker, creative arts therapist, occupational therapist, physician) to respond to the questions: "Why should this patient continue to come here?;" "What additional progress is it reasonable for us to expect in the next few weeks or months?;" What other modalities (e.g., inpatient, outpatient, rehabilitation) might be preferable to day treatment at this time?" Even if the team concludes that "more of the same" is indicated, the *reasoning process* in reaching this conclusion should be traceable.

## REGULATION OF THE MILIEU

After further consideration, Dr. Tuferwun decided to develop a specialized schedule for her program. She hired a group therapist, Ms. Lax, to lead check-in and wrap-up sessions and to coordinate daily activities. Ms. Lax's philosophy was to run meetings in a passive, reflective manner, reasoning that such a "neutral" stance encourages patients actively to seek solutions to their problems, rather than to rely continuously on the staff, thus perpetuating their dependency on the program.

In time, the group began focusing intently on the intimate extragroup relationship that had apparently developed between two members, Dave and Lisa. Dave, a 24-year-old, married man with two children, was admitted to the program because of chronic depression and debilitating alcohol dependence. Lisa, a 22-year-old, single woman, had been admitted for anxiety and self-mutilation. Ms. Lax listened attentively to the developing group process, interpreting the "couple's" seeming exhibitionist qualities and the group's attention to the affair to the exclusion of other issues. Eventually, Dave elected to call off the relationship. Lisa became distraught and angry, and told Dave's wife about the affair. Subsequently, she phoned Dave's employer and informed her of Dave's alcoholism.

### Setting the Ground Rules

By design, the physical and psychological boundaries among members of therapeutic communities are highly permeable. The intimate atmosphere elicits powerful emotions and transferential reactions, creating a substantial risk of behavioral acting out. Extragroup attachments, including sexual relations, frequently develop, and there is a notable tendency for members to gossip about what they have heard or witnessed in the sessions (e.g., Keith-Spiegel & Koocher, 1985; Lakin, 1988; Parker, 1976).

Significantly, this risk of acting out is exacerbated by the relatively diminished influence of milieu personnel over patients in comparison with that of individual therapists. In groups, behavioral contingencies—support versus ostracism, for example—are applied by multiple parties in a reciprocal manner, thus decreasing members' dependence on the leader (Lakin, 1988; Rosenthal, 1987). Further, unlike inpatient groups, partial-hospital patients spend most of their time away from the program, and it is actually beneficial for them to establish and maintain some contact with each other to provide needed support and encouragement. As a result, it is very difficult for milieu leaders to monitor and control patients' extragroup actions.

However, program leaders must establish sufficient ground rules for group and milieu therapy to be successful. At a minimum, they must clarify and accentuate those rules or standards of conduct that are essential for maintaining the very integrity of the group. Any behavior that creates a substantial risk of members' decompensating, dropping out, or losing confidence in each other or the group leader must be addressed. Clearly, breaches of confidentiality and transferential acting out fall into this high-risk category.

Although it is not always possible for milieu personnel to prevent acting out, it is their legal and ethical responsibility to ensure that members recognize and understand the potential negative consequences of such behavior (e.g., Lakin, 1988). This requires program leaders to educate patients—at a level commensurate with their intellectual and emotional development—about the importance of mutual or shared confidentiality, milieu safety, the risks of extragroup relations, and the basics of group process. These admonitions should be repeated and accentuated as necessary, particularly when a violation of the "code" is currently ongoing.

In higher functioning groups, it may be therapeutically appropriate to rely on interpretation and group process to contain acting out (Rosenthal, 1987; Yalom, 1985). However, with a regressed population, education and limit setting are essential components of the leader's repertoire (e.g., Hoge & McLoughlin, 1991). If the goal of partial treatment is to increase adaptation, helping members to avoid the foreseeable negative consequences of their actions directly furthers that goal.

## Confrontational Techniques and Premature Disclosure

The morning after Lisa phoned Dave's employer, the group angrily confronted her at check-in. They accused her of selfishly entering into the relationship in the first place, knowing that Dave was married and that he was emotionally vulnerable because of his drinking. Several members stated that they would not participate in group when Lisa was present because she no longer was trustworthy. In tears, Lisa protested that there were reasons why she did such things, but that she didn't wish to discuss them. The group pressure persisted, but Ms. Lax did not intervene, believing that it was in Lisa's best interest to take responsibility for her actions and to face this maladaptive behavior pattern that she perpetually enacted. Finally, Lisa blurted out that as a child, she had been sexually abused by her uncle, and that she only knew how to relate to men in a sexual manner. She apologized to Dave and the group. Later that night, she cut her wrists in an apparent suicide gesture.

Under certain circumstances, group confrontation can facilitate a member's assumption of responsibility for his or her predicament, and the availability of multiple perspectives can lead to novel and adaptive approaches to problems. However, there is also a dangerous tendency in groups for members to press each other excessively for "genuine" emotion, and to demand congruence between thoughts and actions (Keith-Spiegel & Koocher, 1985; Lakin, 1988). Like a novice therapist, the group may attempt prematurely to bypass a member's psychological defenses to instill quick change. Further, groups are notorious for regulating and reinforcing consensus, and members may behave in an excessively punitive manner toward one who has violated majority tenets (Lakin, 1988).

To the extent that confrontational tactics are appropriate for higher functioning patients, they are frequently contraindicated in vulnerable populations because of the significant risk of decompensation (Galinsky & Schopler, 1977; Parker, 1976). With regressed patients, it is essential for clinicians to attend to issues of "timing, tact, and dosage." The purpose of partial hospitalization and intensive outpatient management is to forestall the need for institutionalization (AAPH, 1991a,b; NAPPH & AAPH, 1990). Thus any technique that precipitates decompensation runs counter to industry standards, and potentially exposes the clinician to malpractice liability.

A program leader must exercise reasonable professional judgment in evaluating a patient's capacity for confrontation, and, if necessary, intervene to shield the patient from excessive group pressure. Further, it is essential to determine whether a patient was unsettled by a session, and to provide the necessary supports to prevent further deterioration. In the above vignette, at the very least, Ms. Lax should have met individually with Lisa after the group to assess whether she was unduly upset by her sudden disclosure. It may have been necessary to contract with her for safety until the next session, arrange for a friend or relative to be with her, or transfer her for a brief inpatient stay.

For purposes of risk management, Ms. Lax should note the circumstances surrounding the disclosure in Lisa's medical record. This should include documentation of the rationale for not intervening in the group process, as well as the fact that she had evaluated Lisa's emotional status before allowing her to leave for the day. As a practical matter, in future litigation, if it wasn't documented, it didn't happen!

### Milieu Safety

During Lisa's convalescence, a new patient, Hank, was transferred to the program on conditional release from the inpatient unit, where he had been involuntarily committed for three months following a violent altercation with his girlfriend. The inpatient psychiatrist petitioned the court for this transfer because Hank was no longer acutely agitated. When Lisa returned to the program, she and Hank became friends and began to spend a lot of time together. Notably, Hank has a documented history of problems with sexual identity, failed interpersonal relationships, and violence toward women. However, he chose not to discuss these issues in group, and Ms. Lax felt it was inappropriate to bring them up before he was ready. A few weeks later, after Lisa turned down his sexual advances, Hank struck her with a lamp, causing severe and permanent injuries. The next day, Hank phoned the program, stating that he would never return.

In recent years, outpatient civil commitment has been increasingly used to provide needed mental health services to dangerous and resistant individuals in the most cost-efficient and least restrictive setting.

However, the use of this commitment scheme poses substantial problems for outpatient programs. In most states, involuntary outpatients must meet the same criteria of "dangerousness" as involuntary inpatients (McCafferty & Dooley, 1990). In Pennsylvania, for example, outpatient commitment is used only as a less restrictive alternative to inpatient commitment for persons who pose a substantial risk of harm to self or others (Pennsylvania Mental Health Procedures Act, 1976).

Mental health professionals have a general ("common-law negligence") duty to provide a reasonably safe environment for the treatment of patients. But, as noted, outpatient and partial-program personnel exercise diminished influence over their patients. This lack of control is increased when courts force hospitals to accept patients who are inappropriate for the available programs, particularly as commitment orders typically contain insufficient information on the patient's history to enable effective treatment planning (Keilitz, 1990). If, under some circumstances, partial-program staff members are prevented from providing a safe environment for their patients, what is their legal and ethical responsibility?

In some states, mental health professionals have a "duty to warn" or "duty to protect" third parties from avoidable harm by a patient (*Tarasoff v. Regents of the Univ. of Calif.*, 1976). This duty may be discharged by warning the intended victim, calling the police, initiating a commitment petition, and so forth. Notably, however, the status of this doctrine is far less certain than most clinicians believe. Some states have rejected the analysis outright (e.g., *Boynton v. Burglass*, 1991), while most others have not had occasion to consider the issue. In some jurisdictions, the duty is triggered only if the patient articulates a specific threat against an identifiable victim (e.g., *Brady v. Hopper*, 1983), which did not happen in the case of Hank and Lisa. In contrast, other states have extended the *Tarasoff* protection to persons who are foreseeably at risk (or in the "zone of danger") for injury by the patient (*Hamman v. County of Maricopa*, 1989). Thus, whether Ms. Lax had a duty under *Tarasoff* to protect Lisa would depend on the law in their jurisdiction.

Notably, there is some question whether the *Tarasoff* rationale would apply at all to a situation like this one. The *Tarasoff* doctrine extends protection to *third parties* who are threatened with harm by a patient. Lisa is not, technically speaking, a "third party," but rather a direct patient of Ms. Lax. Arguably, therefore, Ms. Lax would owe her an increased (or at least different) degree of protection.

Another potential source of accountability stems from the doctrine of "informed consent." Patients have the right to be informed of those risks associated with their treatment that a reasonable person would want to know in deciding whether to consent to that treatment (*Canterbury v. Spence,* 1972). Typically, this doctrine is applied to central aspects of treatment; that is, the patient's diagnosis, treatment methodology, potential benefits and side effects, prognosis with and without treatment, and so on. There is some question as to whether it should apply to the background and characteristics of the patient milieu.

The principle underlying informed consent is that patients have a right to sufficient information in order to anticipate and prepare for what will foreseeably happen to them. Under some circumstances, information related to treatment context should fall into this category. At a minimum, contextual information should rise to a sufficient level to trigger the doctrine once a risky sequence of events has been set in motion. For example, although it may be argued that Lisa had no right to know about Hank's background at the outset, such a right may have developed as their relationship progressed.

As a practical matter, since Hank and Lisa were in the same treatment group, Ms. Lax was in a position to elicit information about Hank's background in an ethical and clinically appropriate manner. Typically, group leaders press or encourage members to discuss their history and reason(s) for seeking treatment with the group. Such disclosure fosters the group process and is also essential to that individual's treatment.

Even if it was appropriate for Ms. Lax to allow Hank to share his past at his own pace, it would still have been possible to intervene in the relationship and divert injury. For example, Ms. Lax could have spoken generally in the group about the dangers of entering into intimate relationships too quickly, without taking sufficient time to get to know the other person. Given many of the current issues facing our patients (AIDS, venereal disease, unwanted pregnancy, domestic violence, etc.), such psychoeducation would be appropriate even in the absence of a specific intra-group relationship.

An additional safety concern is presented by Hank's elopement from the program. Outpatient commitment requires that clinicians exercise a "policing" function (e.g., McCafferty & Dooley, 1990), ensuring the attendance and compliance of recalcitrant patients and informing the courts of violations of the commitment order. This new responsibility may conflict with the therapeutic role. Further, it could expose clinicians to liability, as they are given the front-line, executive function of implementing a court order and protecting the public-at-large.

What is the responsibility of a clinician when a committed patient elopes? At a minimum, the clinician should inform the police and the committing court. Further, he or she should make reasonable efforts to locate the patient, such as calling and writing to the patient's last-known residence and contacting friends, relatives, and employer (without breaching confidentiality). All such efforts should be clearly documented on the patient's chart. Remember, if it isn't written down, it didn't happen.

Additional safety concerns are presented if an assaultive patient remains in the program. For example, if Hank had returned to the partial hospital in his agitated condition, it might have been necessary to use seclusion or restraint, or to transfer him to the inpatient service. It is, therefore, incumbent on partial programs to establish an explicit, workable system or mechanism for handling such crises. As with inpatient care, restraint and seclusion are warranted in "emergencies" to prevent immediate injury to self or others, and the same general guidelines for writing orders and monitoring patients apply (Davidson, Grey, Allende, & Lussier, 1992). If a patient presents an immediate danger, the staff should make reasonable efforts to detain the patient until an appropriate, designated official can evaluate the need to initiate a commitment petition or to order continued restraint.

Generally speaking, given the "intermediate-care" nature of partial treatment, the boundaries between partial programs and outpatient and inpatient services should be flexible (Bendit, 1991; Cuyler, 1991). A patient who is transferred for inpatient stabilization should be able to expect to return to the program, barring unusual circumstances. This gives the message to all of the patients that setbacks are temporary, and that people and relationships do not readily cease to exist.

## CONCLUSION

In the limited space available, we were able to address only the most commonly confronted dilemmas presented in hospital-based partial programs, including program location, specialized scheduling and treatment planning, patient-selection criteria, regulation of group dynamics, and milieu safety. However, the same underlying principles should be applied in resolving the myriad of other legal, ethical, clinical, and administrative issues that are raised by this innovative new class of mental-health-care programs.

## REFERENCES

American Association for Partial Hospitalization. (1991a). *Standards and guidelines for partial hospitalization.* Alexandria, VA: Author.

American Association for Partial Hospitalization. (1991b). *Standards and guidelines for child and adolescent partial hospitalization.* Alexandria, VA: Author.

American Psychiatric Association. (1987). *Diagnostic and statistical manual of mental disorders* (3d ed., rev.). Washington, DC: American Psychiatric Press.

Bach, J. P. (1989). Requiring due care in the process of patient deinstitutionalization: Toward a common law approach to mental health care reform. *Yale Law Journal, 98,* 1153–1172.

Baker, E. L., & McColley, S. (1982). Therapeutic strategies for the aftercare of the schizophrenic: An object relations perspective. *International Journal of Partial Hospitalization, 1,* 119–129.

Bendit, E. A. (1991). If partial-hospital programs come of age: Some caveats. *Psychiatric Hospital, 22,* 77–80.

*Boynton v. Burglass,* 590 So.2d 446 (Fla. App. 1991).

*Brady v. Hopper,* 570 F.Supp. 1333 (D. Colo. 1983), *aff'd,* 751 F.2d 329 (10th Cir. 1984).

*Canterbury v. Spence,* 464 F.2d 772 (D.C. Cir. 1972).

Cuyler, R. N. (1991). The challenge of partial hospitalization in the 1990's. *Psychiatric Hospital, 22,* 47–50.

*Darling v. Charleston Community Memorial Hospital,* 33 Ill.2d 326, 211 N.E.2d 253 (1965), *cert. denied,* 383 U.S. 946 (1966).

Davidson, L., Grey, A., Allende, M., & Lussier, R. G. (1992). Principles for treating aggressive patients in a day hospital: Balancing safety with patient autonomy. *International Journal of Partial Hospitalization, 8,* 1–19.

Doan, R. J., & Petti, T. A. (1990). Patient assessment and treatment planning in child and adolescent partial hospital programs. *Community Mental Health Journal, 26,* 297–308.

Galinsky, M. J., & Schopler, J. H. (1977). Warning: Groups may be dangerous. *Social Work, 22,* 89–94.

*Hamman v. County of Maricopa,* 161 Ariz. 58, 775 P.2d 1122 (1989).

*Helling v. Carey,* 83 Wash.2d 514, 519 P.2d 981 (1974).

Hoge, M. A., Davidson, L., Hill, W. L., Turner, V. E., & Ameli, R. (1992). The promise of partial hospitalization: A reassessment. *Hospital and Community Psychiatry, 43,* 345–354.

Hoge, M. A., Farrell, S. P., Strauss, J. S., & Posner, M. M. (1987). Functions of short-term partial hospitalization in a comprehensive system of care. *International Journal of Partial Hospitalization, 4,* 177–188.

Hoge, M. A., & McLoughlin, K. A. (1991). Group psychotherapy in acute treatment settings: Theory and technique. *Hospital and Community Psychiatry, 42,* 153–158.

Javorsky, J. (1992). Integration of partial hospitalization and inpatient child/adolescent psychiatric units: "A question of continuity of care." *International Journal of Partial Hospitalization, 8,* 65–75.

Joint Commission on Accreditation of Healthcare Organizations. (1991). *Accreditation manual for hospitals* (sec. II). Oakbrook Terrace, IL: Author.

Keilitz, I. (1990). Empirical studies of involuntary outpatient civil commitment: Is it working? *Mental and Physical Disability Law Reporter, 14,* 368–379.

Keith-Spiegel, P., & Koocher, G. P. (1985). *Ethics in psychology: Professional standards and cases.* New York: Random House.

Kennedy, K. L. (1991). Treatment of the borderline patient in partial hospitalization. *Psychiatric Hospital, 22,* 59–67.

Kiser, L. J., Heston, J. D., Millsap, P. A., & Pruitt, D. B. (1991). Treatment protocols in child and adolescent day treatment. *Hospital and Community Psychiatry, 42,* 597–600.

Klar, H., Frances, A., & Clarkin, J. (1982). Selection criteria for partial hospitalization. *Hospital and Community Psychiatry, 33,* 929–933.

Lakin, M. (1988). *Ethical issues in the psychotherapies.* New York: Oxford University Press.

Marlowe, D. B., Tepper, A. M., & Gibbings, E. N. (1992). Clinico-legal issues in partial hospitalization and day treatment. *Comprehensive Mental Health Care, 2,* 201–214.

McCafferty, G., & Dooley, J. (1990). Involuntary outpatient commitment: An update. *Mental and Physical Disability Law Reporter, 14,* 277–287.

Mental Retardation and Community Health Centers Construction Act of 1963, Pub. L. No. 88-164, 77 Stat. 282, *repealed by* Pub. L. No. 97-35 sec. 902 (e)(2)(b), 95 Stat. 560 (1981).

National Association of Private Psychiatric Hospitals and American Association for Partial Hospitalization. (1990). Definition of partial hospitalization. *Psychiatric Hospital, 21,* 89–90.

Parker, R. S. (1976). Ethical and professional considerations concerning high risk groups. *Journal of Clinical Issues in Psychology, 7,* 4–19.

Pennsylvania Mental Health Procedures Act of 1976, PA. Stat. Ann. tit. 50, secs. 7101 *et seq.* (Purdon Supp., 1991).

Rosenthal, L. (1987). *Resolving resistance in group psychotherapy.* Northvale, NJ: Aronson.

Schreer, H. (1988). Therapeutic factors in psychiatric day hospital treatment. *International Journal of Partial Hospitalization, 5,* 307–319.

Tantam, D., & McGrath, G. (1989). Psychiatric day hospitals—another route to institutionalization? *Social Psychiatry and Psychiatric Epidemiology, 24,* 96–101.

*Tarasoff v. Regents of the University of California,* 13 Cal.3d 177, 529 P.2d 533, 118 Cal. Rptr. 129 (1974), *rehearing en banc,* 17 Cal.3d 425, 551 P.2d 334, 131 Cal. Rptr. 14 (1976).

Topp, D. B. (1991). Beyond the continuum of care: Conceptualizing day treatment for children and youth. *Community Mental Health Journal, 27,* 105–113.

Wagner, B. D. (1991). Specialized partial hospitalization for older adults: A clinical description of an intermediate-term program. *Psychiatric Hospital, 22,* 69–76.

Weiss, K. J., & Dubin, W. R. (1982). Partial hospitalization: State of the art. *Hospital and Community Psychiatry, 33,* 923–928.

Yalom, I. D. (1985). *The theory and practice of group psychotherapy* (3d ed.). New York: Basic Books.

# PART IV
# Special Categories

# 11

## AIDS and Psychiatry in the General Hospital
### Legal and Ethical Dilemmas

GOPALAKRISHNA UPADHYA AND
HARVEY BLUESTONE

The acquired immunodeficiency syndrome (AIDS) is a specific group of diseases or conditions that are indicative of severe immunosuppression related to infection with the human immunodeficiency virus (HIV) (Centers for Disease Control [CDC], 1992). AIDS has come to represent the "black death" of the modern era, striking fear into the hearts and minds of people in a way that is reminiscent of the medieval spread of bubonic plague during the 14th century. No other illness in recent history has evoked such public stigmatization, or has been the subject of such political, social, and ethical debate.

Physicians and other health-care workers are not exempt from these fears and so may be hesitant to treat AIDS and HIV-positive patients. Notably, however, the American Medical Association's (AMA) Council on Ethical and Judicial Affairs (1988) recently stated that "a physician may not ethically refuse to treat a patient whose condition is within the physician's current realm of competence solely because the patient is seropositive [for HIV]" (p. 1360). Clarke and Conley (1991), taking note of some clinicians' negative attitudes toward AIDS patients in general, and intravenous drug users and homosexuals in particular, caution that state licensing boards may incorporate this AMA position statement into the legal standard of care. As a result, refusal to treat an AIDS or HIV-positive patient could become grounds for a malpractice action or license revocation.

HIV was isolated and identified as a ribonucleic acid (RNA)–containing retrovirus in 1983 (Barre-Sinoussi et al., 1983). It is both lymphotropic and neurotropic (i.e., infects both lymphatic and neural cells). The virus replicates in these cells, eventually causing cell death. In proliferating, the virus decimates its host, the $T_4$ (helper–inducer) lymphocyte, resulting in defective cellular immunity with cutaneous anergy and an almost pathognomonic reversal of the $T_4$ to $T_8$ (suppressor–cytotoxic) cell ratio (Fauci et al., 1984). This impairment of immunological function allows opportunistic infections and specific neoplasms to develop in HIV-infected persons.

Patients with AIDS and HIV infection present with multiple medical, neurological, psychiatric, and social problems. The immunological breakdown gives rise to severe infections and neoplasms that require vigorous, in-hospital medical care. Further, in addition to immunosuppression, HIV directly affects the central nervous system (CNS) (Price et al., 1988), causing various organic mental syndromes. AIDS and HIV-positive patients have presented with cognitive impairment, language and movement disorders, blindness, mood disorders, psychosis, delirium, and dementia. Additionally, other psychiatric conditions, such as reactive depression, anxiety, panic, and suicidal ideation, may be encountered.

## MANAGEMENT OF AGGRESSIVE SEROPOSITIVE PATIENTS

HIV-infected and AIDS patients retain the personality and social problems that preceded the infection, which is superimposed on the emotional and social issues inherent in homosexuality, drug abuse, promiscuity, and frequent blood transfusions. Borderline and narcissistic character pathology, with chronic dysphoria, affective instability, impaired impulse control, and behavioral acting out, may be present as a premorbid or comorbid condition.

The management difficulties presented by hospitalized seropositive and AIDS patients place great strains on health-care workers. In the first place, workers are concerned about not knowing that a patient in their care is seropositive. As HIV transmission in the workplace has been reported following needle-stick and laceration injuries, there is a pervasive fear of exposure to infected bodily fluids. Thus it is essential that health-care providers follow CDC guidelines in the management of all patients, whether or not their sero status is known.

Psychiatrists may be in a unique position to help primary care-takers confront their fears and anxieties in order to provide optimal treatment for AIDS patients. For example, irrational fears of contagion may result in indirectly punitive behavior toward the patient, causing great distress to both the patient and staff. The following case is illustrative.

**Case 1**

Ramon, age 38, was admitted to the medical service with symptoms of full-blown AIDS. He became increasingly agitated, abusive, and non-compliant with medication and ward routine, and hospital security was called to help restrain him. In response, Ramon threatened to bite the security officer and "give him AIDS." This caused pandemonium on the ward, and an emergency psychiatric consultation was called. On interview, the patient was found to be calm and nonthreatening. He was not psychotic. There was no prior history of psychiatric evaluation or treatment, but he gave a long history of intravenous drug abuse, which presumably was the source of his HIV infection. He also gave a long history of delinquent behavior, including many arrests and two jail sentences. He said he was upset because "I did not get my metha-done this morning. I would have bitten that security officer. There is nothing you can do to me. I'm dying." The patient was fully cognizant of the dangers of his abusive behavior and the consequences of his threat to the security officer. He felt neglected and helpless in the face of his rapidly deteriorating physical condition.

*Discussion of Case 1*

The case of Ramon illustrates many of the difficulties—medical, ethi-cal, and legal—that confront staff members responsible for a danger-ous, terminally ill AIDS patient. Ramon had a long-standing antisocial personality disorder antedating his infection with HIV. Any social constraints that might be instituted (which were ineffective when he was "healthy") were now totally ineffective as he knew that he was dying. The staff felt frustrated, angry, and helpless. Ramon threatened their personal safety, as well as their professional self-image as individuals trained and dedicated to treating individuals with the goal of making them well. The frustration and anger made the situation worse, as the methadone was not promptly given, with almost disastrous results. The psychiatrist needed to help the staff deal with these feelings, so as to diffuse the crisis, and to assist, as needed, in the implementation of restraint, seclusion, or close observation, which required familiarity with applicable laws and policies. The dangerous patient with AIDS is an extreme example of the need for psychiatric intervention, with skill in assessment and interpersonal interaction and knowledge of forensic issues.

Psychiatrists are being increasingly called upon to evaluate AIDS patients' mental capacity to participate meaningfully in the clinical decision-making process. Given the nature of CNS involvement in AIDS, resulting in various forms of organic mental syndromes such as delirium and AIDS dementia complex, issues of competency, capacity to give informed consent, and decisions concerning life-sustaining measures and DNR (Do Not Resuscitate) orders take on new meaning. Conflicting public attitudes and rapidly changing laws governing the care of HIV-infected persons serve to complicate these issues.

## PARTNER AND PUBLIC HEALTH SERVICES NOTIFICATION

The AIDS epidemic has created some of the most difficult and controversial ethical and legal problems concerning confidentiality (Dickens, 1990). Frequently, the ethical obligation to maintain patient confidentiality directly conflicts with the need to protect unsuspecting sexual and needle-sharing partners. Since 1988 the CDC has made the existence of partner-notification programs a precondition for the granting of federal funds to the states from its HIV prevention program. Notification programs have also been endorsed by the Institute of Medicine of the National Academy of Sciences (1988) and a Presidential Commission on the HIV epidemic.

The Council on Ethical and Judicial Affairs of the AMA (1988) reminds physicians that they are ethically obligated to respect the rights of privacy and confidentiality of AIDS patients and seropositive individuals. However, where there is no statute that mandates or prohibits the reporting of seropositive individuals who present a danger to others, the AMA recommends that the physician take the following steps: (1) attempt to persuade the infected patient to cease endangering the third party; (2) if persuasion fails, notify authorities; and (3) if the authorities take no action, notify the endangered third party.

The American Psychiatric Association (APA) (1988, p. 541) has issued the following AIDS policy statement on confidentiality and disclosure:

> Notification of Third Parties: In situations where a physician has received convincing clinical information that the patient is infected with HIV, the physician should advise and work with the patient either to obtain the patient's agreement to terminate behavior that places other persons at risk of infection or to notify identifiable individuals who may be at continuing risk of exposure. If a patient refuses to agree to change his or her behavior or to notify the person(s) at risk or the physician has good reason to believe that the patient has failed to or is unable to comply with this agreement, it is *ethically permissible* for the physician to notify an identifiable person who the physician believes is in danger of contracting the virus (italics added).

As of 1990, only two states had imposed on physicians a legal duty to warn spouses that they were at risk for HIV infection. Several states passed legislation granting physicians the privilege of immunity from liability for warning sexual and needle-sharing partners, thus freeing them from liability whether or not they issued such warnings. In some states, including New York, these warnings may not include revealing the identity of the source of the threat of infection.

It is important to note that clinical AIDS has been a reportable condition in all 50 states since 1983. Yet, by 1991, only a few states had mandatory reporting of seropositive individuals. Most state laws, as well as the position statements of the AMA and APA, involve *permissive* disclosure of *future* risks of infection. Consider the nuances of the following three case vignettes.

## CASE EXAMPLES

### Case 2

Ian is a 35-year-old man who was recently diagnosed with AIDS after a brief bout of pneumonia. He probably became infected with the virus during a two-year period of intravenous drug use, which had started approximately four years earlier. He has been married for three years, and although his wife knows of his history of drug abuse, she has never suspected that he was sharing needles with other drug abusers.

Over the years, the couple has used condoms, as well as a diaphragm with spermicidal cream, for birth control. The patient reports that since his HIV-positive diagnosis, he has attempted to use condoms all the time. However, "slips" still occur. He refuses to tell his wife of his diagnosis, fearing that she will abandon him, and says that he would kill himself if she were to leave him.

### Case 3

Adrian, a 28-year-old homosexual man with a diagnosis of borderline personality disorder, was originally referred for psychiatric treatment when he made a serious suicide attempt following the breakup of a one-year relationship. He was diagnosed HIV-positive six months earlier, after a brief period of fever, weight loss, and diarrhea. In the past, Adrian had multiple sexual partners and he frequented bathhouses. He also engaged in heavy nonintravenous (marijuana and cocaine) drug abuse. In addition, there is a possible history of homosexual prostitution to help finance his drug habit.

Adrian recently became involved in a serious, monogamous relationship. He and his partner do not use condoms, having assured each other of their seronegative status for HIV. Adrian fears rejection by his lover if he admits his seropositivity, and he thus informed his therapist of his intention to drop out of treatment if the therapist attempted to notify the partner. Furthermore, he threatened that he would seek revenge by infecting other unsuspecting individuals.

### Case 4

Tatiana is a 30-year-old woman who had been an intravenous drug abuser for 10 years and is now receiving treatment in a drug rehabilitation program as an evening outpatient. She has been drug-free for over a year, but was recently found to be seropositive for HIV. Tatiana works during the day in a neighborhood food market, and is supporting her 65-year-old disabled mother and her five-year-old son. Over the past 10 years, Tatiana has had three steady relationships with men, two of whom used drugs with her. Tatiana does not wish to reveal her HIV status to any of her previous boyfriends, as she fears that such information would circulate through the neighborhood, resulting in the loss of her job and social ostracism.

*Discussion of Cases*

These cases illustrate the complicated, and often conflicting, roles that health-care professionals must assume with regard to AIDS patients: (1) the role of clinician, with the goals of treating the patient and managing the therapeutic relationship; (2) the role of professional, with the goal of maintaining client privacy and confidentiality; and (3) the role of protector of the public-at-large, with the goal of warning potential victims of harm. Given that most state notification laws and professional position statements contain permissive language, it is necessary for clinicians to exercise professional discretion in resolving apparent conflicts among these roles.

The case of Ian primarily implicates the psychiatrist's treatment role. It concerns the right of a spouse or significant other to know of HIV infection, versus the patient's fear of resulting abandonment. Ideally, the therapist should explore this underlying fear further, and attempt to help the couple to achieve a more open communication and to sustain the relationship. Given that the marriage appears to be stable and the patient is apparently monogamous, it is ethically sound to approach the problem—at least in the short run—as a therapeutic issue.

If the therapeutic approach fails, it may become necessary at some point to contact the wife or local health department. However, the therapist must then bear in mind the patient's potential to commit suicide if his wife were to leave him. It would not be unusual for a person to become extremely despondent after learning of HIV infection and then losing a loved one.

The case of Adrian also illustrates the underlying fear of rejection following partner notification. However, in this case, the stability of the relationship is questionable, and the likelihood of contact with multiple parties in the future is higher. The patient may also pose a threat to the community-at-large because of his acting-out tendencies and his threatening remarks to the therapist. Here, the likelihood of success of a therapeutic approach is minimal, and the public health role assumes prominence.

In the case of Tatiana, the fear is related to the possible loss of her job and social abandonment. The risk of future infection by her is minimized because she does not currently have a sexual partner, and she is apparently drug-free. From a public health perspective, the only advantage of partner notification here would be to prevent further spread of the disease by her previous boyfriends, assuming that they are also infected. Because the public health role is lessened, the professional ethical duty of confidentiality assumes greater prominence. Tatiana's fears of neighborhood stigma are probably legitimate, and it may be that disclosure will do more harm than good. In this case, the therapist may wish to help her to inform her past boyfriends (perhaps anonymously), without involving public agencies. Here, discretion may be able to go hand-in-hand with public safety.

In the cases of Ian and Tatiana, failure on the part of the clinician to disclose seropositivity would not appear to violate professional ethical mandates. For example, the APA position statement permits notification to protect individuals at "continuing" risk. In these cases, the infection, if any, has likely already taken place.

It is important to note that clinicians should not assume that patients engaged in high-risk behavior fully understand the risks involved. An educational, directive therapy may be warranted (Kleinman, 1991). Similarly, when a patient engages in behavior that may harm others, the first step should be to attempt to understand the conscious or unconscious motivations directing the behavior. Such motivation might include an attempt to deny the reality of the fatal condition, transferential acting out, a wish for revenge, a lack of impulse control, or an inability to consider the perspective of others. The therapist should attempt to persuade the patient to look at these aberrant behaviors more rationally, and to help the patient change these dangerous behaviors, by using the leverage and pressure of the positive therapeutic alliance. Only when such attempts fail, or appear futile, should the therapist resort to other measures.

# REFERENCES

American Medical Association Council on Ethical and Judicial Affairs. (1988). Ethical issues involved in the growing AIDS crisis. *JAMA, 259,* 1360–1361.

American Psychiatric Association. (1988). AIDS policy: Confidentiality and disclosure. *American Journal of Psychiatry, 145,* 541.

Barre-Sinoussi, F., Chermann, J. C., Rey, F., Nugeyre, M. T., Chamaret, S., Frerest, J., Daugnet, C., Axler-Blin, C., Vezinet-Brern, F., Rouzioux, C., Rosenbaum, N., & Montagnier, L. (1983). Isolation of a T-lymphotropic retrovirus from a patient at risk for acquired immune deficiency syndrome (AIDS). *Science, 220,* 868–871.

Centers for Disease Control. (1992, January). *HIV/AIDS surveillance report* (pp. 1–22). Washington, DC: Author.

Clarke, O., & Conley, R. (1991). The duty to attend upon the sick. *JAMA, 266,* 2876–2877.

Dickens, B. (1990). AIDS: Confidentiality and the duty to warn. In L. Gostin (Ed.), *AIDS and the health care system* (pp. 98–114). New Haven, CT: Yale University Press.

Fauci, A. S., Macher, A. M., Longo, D. L., Lane, H. C., Rook, A. H., Masur, H., & Gelmann, E. P. (1984). Acquired immunodeficiency syndrome: Epidemiologic, clinical, immunologic, and therapeutic considerations. *Annals of Internal Medicine, 100,* 92–106.

Institute of Medicine of the National Academy of Sciences. (1988). *Confronting AIDS: Update 1988.* Washington, DC: National Academy Press.

Kleinman, I. (1991). Ethical and legal considerations in psychotherapy. *Canadian Journal of Psychiatry, 36,* 121–122.

Price, R. W., Brew, B., Sidtis, J., Rosenbaum, M., Scheck, A. C., & Cleary, P. (1988). The brain and AIDS: Central nervous system HIV-I infection and AIDS dementia complex. *Science, 239,* 586–591.

# 12

## Psychiatric Training, Supervision, and Shared Responsibility
### Some Forensic Concerns

RICHARD ROSNER

The following observations, remarks, suggestions, and recommendations are meant to raise issues, stimulate constructive reflection, and offer a particular viewpoint regarding some forensic concerns that relate to psychiatric training, supervision, and shared responsibility. The goal is to encourage thought, not necessarily to advocate for any particular position. The cases are set in an imaginary state, so that all supposed facts and opinions should be regarded as illustrations of principles and problems; they are not meant to be directly applicable to the actual state in which the reader may practice. One should not assume that his or her current policies and procedures must be changed immediately, or, on the other hand, that they are necessarily correct as they stand, but should consider the laws in the individual state and the applicability of this discussion to his or her specific hospital, practice, and circumstances.

## THE PROBLEMS

### Illustrative Cases

*Case A*

It is 4:30 P.M. on Friday afternoon of the third week in July, three weeks into the start of the work of the most recently hired group of interns. Mrs. A. advises the intern assigned to her case that she wants to leave the hospital immediately. The intern is reluctant to let her go. She volunteers to sign the same type of form that she signed on one of her seven prior admissions, to signify that she is leaving against medical advice. The intern had spoken with his supervisor a few days earlier about the fact that Mrs. A., who had voluntarily admitted herself for treatment of her depression, had just begun to show a bit more energy, probably the first signs that her antidepressant was working. Now the intern is worried that Mrs. A.'s desire to leave may indicate a concealed intention to act on the very suicidal ideas for which she initially sought help. Concerned as to what to do, he calls his supervisor.

*Case B*

Mr. B.'s nurse advises the resident that Mr. B. is glaring threateningly and shouting obscenities at any patients or staff members who approach him. She suggests that he may need to be medicated involuntarily to reduce the risk that he will act violently against another patient or a staff member. The resident disagrees. Mr. B. has repeatedly refused medications and the resident is concerned that forcing him to take them will undermine the fragile therapeutic relationship that he is just beginning to establish with Mr. B. However, he says that he will contact his supervisor and be guided by the advice that he will receive.

*Case C*

Ms. C. is HIV seropositive, most likely as a result of her past use of shared needles to self-administer intravenous drugs. She is an employee of the hospital, where she works in the billing department. She recently moved into the neighborhood in order to be close to her job. She is being treated in the hospital's psychiatric clinic in the outpatient department. In addition to the fact that she receives clinical services at a reduced rate because of her employee status, the hospital is the closest care provider to her new home. At the start of therapy, she explained that she was reluctant to speak freely about her problems because she feared that her chart records might be seen by other employees who know her, and she worried that information about her might "leak" from the hospital to the community. When her therapist explained that all of her records were confidential, she accused him of being naive and demanded that he take special precautions with her chart, so that no one else could see it. She threatened to sue the therapist if anyone were to find out about her HIV seropositivity. After learning from the hospital administrator that no separate set of medical chart records can be created and stored independently of all other records specifically to meet the concerns of any one patient, the therapist decided to discuss the matter at his next supervisory session.

*Discussion*

Psychiatric training, supervision, and shared responsibility in the general hospital entail forensic concerns. Multiple interested parties have potentially conflicting legal rights and responsibilities. The parties may include some or all of the following:

- The general hospital, as a corporate entity
- The Nursing Department, which has its own administrative, professional practice, and academic interests
- The Social Service Department
- The Department of Psychiatry as one among many administrative subunits of the general hospital
- The medical school, with which the Department of Psychiatry may be affiliated
- The ward chiefs of the individual subunits into which the general hospital is divided
- The team leader of the health-care service-delivery group
- The individual supervisor
- The individual supervisee (e.g., intern, resident, fellow)
- The individual patient.

Training and supervision take place in a complex network of administrative and professional hierarchical relationships; it is an error to think that the supervisor and supervisee are free to function as they may mutually agree to do.

Matters are further complicated because forensic concerns are only one of many constraints on the practice of training, supervision, and shared responsibility. Among the others, sometimes confused with forensic concerns, are the following:

- Morality: what is morally right may or may not coincide with what is legally permissible or impermissible.
- Prudence: what is best for any one of the many interested parties enumerated above is not necessarily the same as what is legal or illegal.
- Economics: what is least expensive may be illegal, whereas what is most costly may be legally mandatory.
- Religion: what is forbidden by one's personal religion may be required by law; what is required by one's personal religion may be forbidden by law.
- Obedience to authority in general: doing what a supervisor has directed does not absolve a supervisee from legal responsibility; the Nazi claims that they were "following orders" were not exculpatory at the Nuremberg war crimes trials.
- Personal opinions/biases/tastes: idiosyncratic inclinations that are appropriate or harmless in private life may be inconsistent with legal obligations.

The general guideline for supervisors to keep in mind is that they are personally legally responsible for the professional practices of their supervisees. The legal doctrine of respondeat superior (i.e., the principal is responsible for the agent) is generally applicable to the supervisor–supervisee relationship.

Supervisors may have assumed legal responsibilities unwittingly; they may not know that they are potentially liable for the professional practice errors of their supervisees. This is a common occurrence. A supervisor may have been told of the existence of a hospital manual of policies and procedures, but not have been directed to the section of the manual addressing supervisory liability issues. A supervisor may have been advised that he or she can confer with his or her own immediate superior or the general hospital administrator about any questions, but not know enough to ask about liability. A supervisor may erroneously believe that he or she is immune from legal responsibility for a supervisee's professional practice. However, ignorance of the law is not an excuse.

The general guideline for supervisees to keep in mind is that they are also personally legally responsible for their professional practice; they cannot successfully transfer full responsibility for their conduct to another interested party. Some interns, residents, and fellows erroneously believe that the general hospital will be liable for their professional activities, and may lack an understanding of the law that might motivate them to seek competent supervision.

Both the supervisor and the supervisee need to be clear that shared responsibility refers to two matters: (1) their mutual decision-making processes regarding patient care, and (2) their joint legal responsibility for the care that is provided. Their shared authority entails shared accountability. In addition to being motivated by altruistic reasons to cooperate, they have prudent reasons to work together. To borrow from Benjamin Franklin, if they do not hang together, they will surely be hanged separately.

As a practical matter, it is important to both supervisor and supervisee to document their supervisory meetings. Adequate documentation may constitute the best evidence in their defense against any malpractice charges. A written record substantiates the fact that, at a minimum, some supervision actually took place, consistent with the supervisor's obligation to provide it and the supervisee's obligation to obtain it.

Confusion abounds regarding records of supervision: Who should maintain the record, the supervisor or the supervisee? What should be included in the record, and what should be omitted? Should notes be brief or extensive? Where should the record be kept, on the patient's chart or separately? Are supervisory notes protected by doctor–patient confidentiality, and, if so, who can waive that confidentiality (the supervisor, the supervisee, the patient)? Who can have access to supervisory notes (the hospital administration, the ward secretary, the file clerks in the hospital record room, the patient)?

Hospitals and individual supervisors vary in their answers to these questions. Common practices include:

1. Having the supervisor sign the supervisee's periodic chart notes to indicate that they were reviewed. This requires the supervisor

to come to the hospital because the chart cannot be taken from the premises, and this may be considered a burden by some supervisors. It is the most minimal written evidence of supervision that can be demonstrated, but will be of little value in a professional liability suit.

2. Having the supervisor or supervisee record on the chart the bare fact that a supervision session occurred. This is the second most minimal evidence of supervision and also is of little value in a malpractice case.

3. Having the supervisor or supervisee summarize the conclusions reached during the supervisory session. This begins to address the substance of the supervision, providing the first real basis for a legal defense against liability claims.

4. Having the supervisor or supervisee summarize the main issues discussed, the clinical data considered relevant to those issues, the reasoning processes applied to those issues, and the conclusions reached during the supervisory session. This constitutes an adequate record of the supervisory process for medical–legal purposes. It establishes that alternatives were considered, demonstrating that professional medical judgments were made. Wrong choices among alternative professional judgments are not themselves evidence of malpractice, but, failure to consider relevant issues, data, and alternative conclusions may lead to professional liability, on the grounds that evidence is lacking that any professional medical judgment actually took place.

The supervisory sessions are, in some respects, a special class of consultations obtained by the principal treating physician (the supervisee) from an experienced colleague (the supervisor). Obtaining such a consultation is one of the ways in which a practitioner can establish that diligent efforts were made to provide appropriate care for the patient. Good records of the supervisory process help to protect the principal treating physician (the supervisee) from liability, and also help to protect the supervisor by documenting that adequate supervision was provided.

As with all medical records, it can be argued that anything can and will be used against the supervisor and supervisee in the course of malpractice litigation. Some physicians go so far as to suggest that no records be kept, so that nothing can be used against them. However, that position ignores the fact that by removing the record as a sword in the hands of the complainant-patient, one is also removing the record as a shield in the hands of the defendant-doctor. It is better to have adequate records than minimal records. It is foolhardy to have no records whatsoever.

The supervisory session is protected by doctor–patient confidentiality. The right to insist on or waive that confidentiality belongs to the patient. The written data about the supervisory sessions are similarly protected as part of a patient's medical records. But hospital chart records are seen by so many people that the word "confidential" approaches ·is misleading. Among those to whom these records are available are the ward secretaries, the record-room file clerks, the health-care utilization reviewers, the medical insurance auditors, inspectors from hospital accreditation organizations, and inspectors from internship and residency training accreditation organizations, as well as other members of the treatment team. The supervisor and supervisee should be aware of how many others will have access to a written supervisory report that is part of the patient's hospital chart.

The argument that supervisory notes should be kept apart from the patient's hospital chart is based on the fact that so many, perhaps too many, people can look at that chart. However, supervision is not a secret that only the supervisor and the supervisee should know about. The supervisory records may be confidential, but they are not secret. The records of all other consultations are incorporated into the patient's chart, and there is no compelling reason why the supervisory consultations should not also be part of the chart. A further argument against keeping the supervisory notes separately is that it creates a considerable secondary filing and storage burden. Also, a separate set of records increases the risk of lost records. As a practical matter, it is more convenient to make the supervisory records part of the patient's hospital chart.

Who is in charge of the patient's care? Is the supervisee free to regard the supervisory session as a consultation that he or she can either heed or ignore? Is the supervisor powerless to ensure that his or her sage counsel will be implemented? Who is in charge when there is shared responsibility? There are a variety of answers, depending on the specific type of supervisory relationship.

1. In some relationships, such as that of an intern (supervisee) and his or her immediately superior resident (supervisor), it may be understood that the intern (supervisee) has limited independent authority and that the resident (supervisor) can countermand and initiate orders. The ward chief has the same authority to overrule everyone under his or her administrative authority, for example, all the interns and all the residents. The chairperson of the Department of Psychiatry has the same authority over all of the interns, residents, and ward chiefs. This is a quasi-military hierarchy of authority, a chain of command from the top to the bottom.

2. In some relationships—such as that of a teacher and student, senior practitioner and junior practitioner, or experienced consultant and less experienced trainee—there are a moral authority and a persuasive authority (the ability, based on greater knowledge and experience, to convince the supervisee of the value of decisions recommended by the supervisor), but there is no absolute power to override the supervisee's decisions and intervene in a patient's care. This second type of supervisory relationship commonly exists between the hospital's part-time, unsalaried, clinical faculty members and the interns, residents, and fellows, who are trainees. In extreme situations, this second type of supervisor has the option of directly contacting a supervisor of the first type. Thus the second type of supervisor, who lacks direct authority, can make certain that someone with actual power to initiate and countermand the supervisee's orders can intervene, taking the control of a patient's care away from the supervisee, and in this way can exert direct influence on patient care.

While both types of supervisors share responsibility for the care delivered to patients, their direct authority to control that care is not the same. Both types of supervisors can be implicated in professional liability suits, but the difference in their degree of direct control over a patient's care may be relevant to the court's apportionment of liability in any given case. However, no supervisor should mistake the possibility of being regarded as only partially liable for the errors of a supervisee as the equivalent of having no substantial liability: the risk cannot be completely avoided. Further, regardless of whether or not he or she is actually found responsible in a malpractice case, the supervisor is vulnerable to the nuisance, the stress, and the burdens of the malpractice suit itself as it drags on, seemingly interminably, through the court processes.

Both the supervisor and supervisee share, in varying degrees, the authority and accountability for the patient's care. The list of persons sharing therapeutic responsibility may be long. In the extreme case, the student social worker has a supervisor, the student nurse has a supervisor, the medical student has a supervisor, the intern has a supervisor, and the first-, second-, and third-year residents all have supervisors. The patient is unlikely to know how many are on the treatment team. Who is responsible for telling the patient that an extended treatment team exists?

In some hospitals, while the salaried staff is visibly present, the part-time, voluntary, unsalaried, clinical faculty is essentially invisible. The clinical supervisor and supervisee may meet regularly, but outside of the view and awareness of the patient. Is the patient's right to informed consent being respected if he or she is never told that the supervisor shares responsibility for the patient's care? Is the patient's right to confidentiality being respected if he or she is never told that a third party, the supervisor, is privy to the patient's communications?

The inpatients on a hospital ward usually see that a team of doctors, nurses, social workers, and clerical staff members is taking care of the ward's patients. However, the patients in the hospital's outpatient department may not see the team of care givers, and they may not even know that the team exists. The patient may believe that he or she has entered into a dyadic, confidential relationship with the outpatient-clinic doctor, when the truth is that a host of third parties is privy to almost all of the patient's communications. Is this almost-never-revealed, diffusion of access to the patient's records consistent with the informed consent to treatment that is required by law? Is it a breach of confidentiality to reveal the patient's communications or to permit access to the patient's records to that host of third parties? Does the patient have the right to know the names of the persons to whom his or her records are available and of those who are sharing responsibility for his or her care?

Generally, the patient is entitled to know who the care givers are. In most hospitals, it is thought to be common knowledge that a health-care team exists, and that information about the patient is exchanged freely among members of the treatment team. Further, it is thought to be common knowledge that medical students, interns, residents, and fellows are supervised. But even if such information were commonly known to most patients, there might be some who are not aware of it. Further, it is one thing to know that a student doctor, student nurse, student social worker, intern, resident, and fellow are being supervised, but it is quite another to know exactly what the nature of the supervision is and who is providing it. Informed consent to treatment entails knowing who the members of the treatment team are—all of them. Confidentiality grants the patient the right to determine who will have access to information about his or her care; that right is not meaningful if the patient is not advised as to what persons in the hospital will have such access routinely.

The patient should be specifically told that a health-care team exists, rather than it being assumed that such information is common knowledge. The patient also should be told that supervision is provided to all students, interns, residents, and fellows. If the patient asks, the individual supervisee should furnish the name of the supervisor and basic information about the supervisory process—for example, that all supervisees have supervisors, that supervision is regularly scheduled, that the goals of supervision include enhancing the patient's well-being, and that the supervisor is a more experienced, practicing clinician. The patient should be informed, as well, that hospital clerks, hospital administrators, and hospital-care auditors will have access to the hospital's records containing information about the patient. How to be candid about these matters without causing needless anxiety is an interpersonal skill that must be fostered.

In some instances of supervision, one has a case of the blind leading the blind. The supervisors may be insufficiently familiar with forensic psychiatric issues to be competent to teach the supervisees about those issues. Supervisors are most often selected because of their clinical skills, rather than for their familiarity with psychiatric–legal matters. How can a supervisor ascertain whether a supervisee has complied with the informed-consent requirements regarding patient care if the supervisor is unfamiliar with those requirements? What is needed is a systematic effort to educate the educators. Such an effort should include written materials, oral presentations, and the availability of special second-level supervision and consultation on forensic issues. The written materials, at minimum, should include the hospital policies and procedures manual, with special attention to those portions that relate to legal concerns. The oral presentations should be given either by an attorney or by a psychiatrist experienced in forensic issues. An attorney may be seen as a more authoritative figure by the psychiatric supervisory staff, but also may be perceived as lacking an understanding of clinical realities. A psychiatrist experienced in forensic issues may be more readily accepted as understanding the clinical issues to which the law applies. This should be part of a continuing educational effort. Just as the supervisee needs to be able to seek advice from the supervisor regarding the application of therapeutic principles to the specific patients' cases, so the clinical supervisors need to be able to consult forensic experts regarding the application of the legal principles to the specific patients' cases.

While it is beyond the scope of this chapter to address the details of the psychiatric–legal training that should be provided to the supervisory staff, a brief outline is appropriate. If it is too costly to furnish each supervisor with a basic book on psychiatric–legal issues, at minimum, supervisors should be given a list of recommended readings on the clinical applications of forensic psychiatry. They should be trained to organize psychiatric–legal cases in a format that facilitates their understanding of those cases. And they should be familiar with the organizational framework used by forensic psychiatrists.

1. What is the specific psychiatric–legal issue to be considered? For example, is the issue informed consent, confidentiality, malpractice?
2. What are the legally specified criteria that determine how the issue will be decided? For example, to establish malpractice liability, the legal criteria may be recalled by the mnemonic of "the four Ds": Damages to the patient, directly due to the actions or inactions of the responsible professionals, who had a professional duty to the patient, and who were found to be Deviant/Deficient/Derelict/Delinquent in the performance of their professional duties when compared with the standard for professional practice.

3. What are the clinical data that are relevant to the legally specific criteria? For example, was the patient actually informed about the risk of tardive dyskinesia before being started on neuroleptic medications?

4. What reasoning process was used by the doctor in formulating an opinion on the psychiatric–legal issue? For example, has the doctor shown that the clinical data, as applied to the specific legal criteria, support the resolution of the issue in a manner consistent with his or her opinion?

## SOME SOLUTIONS

### The Cases Revisited

*Case A*

The supervisor explains that although Mrs. A. voluntarily entered the hospital, as a voluntary patient in that state she is not free to leave without permission. Although the patient may sign a form indicating that she chose to leave against medical advice, that form will not protect the members of the treatment team from a malpractice suit if they permit Mrs. A. to leave when they know, or should have known, that she is dangerous to herself. The supervisor advises the intern to tell Mrs. A. that she may not leave until the doctors have had sufficient time to evaluate whether she is a risk to herself. He explains to the intern that the hospital administrator should be so advised and that the hospital security office should be notified (in case the patient attempts to leave without permission). He further explains that it may be necessary to petition the court to convert Mrs. A.'s status from voluntary to involuntary, and that it will be necessary to inform the agency that is charged with the protection of the legal rights of detained mental patients that the patient is being held against her will.

The first psychiatric–legal issue is whether this particular voluntary patient should be permitted to leave the hospital or should be converted to involuntary status. The relevant legal criteria in that state for nonvoluntary hospitalization include the fact that a person's mental illness so impairs his or her judgment that he or she cannot recognize the need for in-hospital treatment or that the person is dangerous to himself or herself or to others. In applying the clinical data to the legal criteria, it is noted that since Mrs. A. had recently been voicing suicidal ideas, her increased energy is insufficient improvement to justify her release. She is still likely to be a risk to herself and she appears to meet the criteria for retention as an involuntary patient. The reasoning process is that set forth here: applying the clinical data to the legal criteria to support the resolution of the issue in favor of not permitting Mrs. A. to leave the hospital.

*Case B*

The resident's supervisor explains that, if the resident believes that Mr. B. is so dangerous that an emergency exists, he can medicate Mr. B. directly without the patient's consent. However, the supervisor also explains that if Mr. B. is not an "emergency," then there are two options: first, the resident can continue to work with Mr. B. and attempt over time to convince him to take medication, and second, the court may be asked to review the matter, and if Mr. B. is found incompetent to make medication decisions, the court has the power to direct that he receive medication involuntarily.

The first psychiatric–legal issue is whether the patient can be medicated involuntarily. The legal criteria in that state for immediate involuntary medication include the fact that an emergency must exist. In this instance, the clinical data indicate that Mr. B. is shouting obscenities and glaring threateningly, but not that he has specifically threatened to harm anyone (although he scares the other patients) or gestured as though to hurt anyone. In applying the data to the criteria, it is seen that Mr. B. is not an "emergency" and cannot be medicated involuntarily at present.

The second psychiatric–legal issue is whether Mr. B. is competent to refuse medications. The legal criteria in that state address whether there is a reasonable and rational ground for refusing the proposed medication. No relevant clinical data are available, because no one has successfully inquired as to why Mr. B. does not want to take medications, although he has repeatedly stated that he does not wish to do so. In the absence of relevant data, there is no way to support a claim that Mr. B. is not competent to refuse medicine. The resident is advised to explore in great detail Mr. B.'s reticence regarding medications. More information than is currently available would be needed if Mr. B. ever were to be taken to court, found incompetent, and directed to take medication.

## Case C

The supervisor explains that some of Ms. C.'s fears are realistic. There is no way to be absolutely certain that an employee who knows Ms. C. might not have access to her medical chart. Further, even though it should not be done, there is no way to be absolutely certain that such an employee might not "leak" the information. If such a leak were to occur, the hospital, the therapist, and the supervisor might be sued for not taking sufficient steps to protect Ms. C.'s confidentiality. The supervisor suggests that Ms. C. be advised that her confidential communications might be more completely protected at a treatment facility at which she is not employed and that is located in a neighborhood in which she does not reside. After full discussion of the possible risks to confidentiality, if Ms. C. wishes to remain in treatment with her current therapist at the hospital clinic, the chart notes should reflect that this matter was discussed in supervision and with Ms. C., and that she freely chose to provide her informed consent to the limited risk of an information leak by remaining in her current therapeutic relationship.

The first psychiatric–legal issue is whether the hospital, the therapist, and the supervisor might be answerable to malpractice charges for failure to preserve Ms. C.'s confidential communications. Malpractice legal criteria in that state include deviation from the professional standard of performance of one's professional obligations to a patient to whom one owes a professional duty, such that damages to the patient directly result from that deviant performance. In view of the patient's status as an employee who can be seen by other employees entering and leaving the hospital's psychiatric outpatient clinic, the risk that other employees will know that she is seeking psychiatric services is real. Although no employee is supposed to look at any patient's chart except in the performance of official duties, it is possible that some other employee might inappropriately look at Ms. C.'s chart. Further, although gossip about any patient is inappropriate, it is possible that data about Ms. C. could leak from one employee to another and then into the community. These events are not likely to happen, but they could. Failure to address this risk with Ms. C. and to assist her in determining how best to protect her interests might be the basis of a liability suit, if the leak were to take place and if Ms. C. were to suffer damages as a result.

The second psychiatric–legal issue relates to informed consent. With a competent patient, a review of the risks and benefits of the proposed treatment and of no treatment, prior to beginning that treatment, is a prerequisite to obtaining informed consent, according to the laws of that state. Failure to obtain a competent patient's voluntary informed consent to a proposed treatment would constitute grounds for a malpractice suit; it would be a deviation from the standard of professional care. By carefully discussing the risks of the possible leak of confidential communication and the benefits of a low-cost, geographically convenient treatment opportunity, and documenting that discussion, the chart records will support a claim that Ms. C. provided informed consent to continuing in treatment at the hospital's psychiatric clinic, should she choose to do so.

## CONCLUSIONS

No single chapter can raise, let alone resolve, the full range of psychiatric–legal issues that will be encountered in the processes of psychiatric training, supervision, and shared responsibility. In this discussion, an effort has been made to present examples of clinical case problems, and to give possible solutions to those problems; to raise questions, and to provide possible answers to those questions; and to stress that awareness of the possibility of forensic concerns is the best protection against entrapment in those concerns.

## REFERENCES

Brooks, A. (1974). *Law, psychiatry and the mental health system.* Boston, MA: Little, Brown.

Curran, W., McGarry, A., & Petty, C. (1980). *Modern legal medicine, psychiatry and forensic science.* Philadelphia, PA: F. A. Davis.

Golding, M. (1975). *Philosophy of law.* Englewood Cliffs, NJ: Prentice-Hall.

Grilliot, H. (1983). *Introduction to law and the legal system.* Boston, MA: Houghton Mifflin.

Rosner, R. (Ed.). (1982). *Critical issues in American psychiatry and the law.* Springfield, IL: Charles C. Thomas.

Rosner, R. (Ed.). (1985). *Critical issues in American psychiatry and the law* (Vol. 2). New York: Plenum.

Rosner, R. (Ed.). (1993). *Principles and practice of forensic psychiatry.* New York: Chapman and Hall.

Rosner, R., & Harmon, R. (Eds.). (1989a). *Criminal court consultation.* New York: Plenum.

Rosner, R., & Harmon, R. (Eds.). (1989b). *Correctional psychiatry.* New York: Plenum.

Rosner, R., & Schwartz, H. (Eds.). (1987). *Geriatric psychiatry and the law.* New York: Plenum.

Rosner, R., & Schwartz, H. (Eds.). (1989). *Juvenile psychiatry and the law.* New York: Plenum.

Rosner, R., & Weinstock, R. (Eds.). (1990). *Ethical practice in psychiatry and the law.* New York: Plenum.

# 13

## The Impaired
## Health Professional
### Legal and Ethical Issues

ROBERT L. SADOFF AND
JULIE B. SADOFF

A "professional" may be considered one who professes an open and public declaration of learning or skill, thereby eliciting expectations from others. By virtue of title, a professional is recognized as an authority and entitled to certain privileges or advantages. By virtue of license, a professional is certified to perform specific functions and earns certain rights or legal entitlements. By virtue of status, a professional stands in a position of authority and incurs responsibility and accountability.

A physician or health professional clearly meets these criteria. The practice of medicine is a privilege, since no one has the right to practice without the necessary qualifications of learning and skill. Once those qualifications are met, a physician obtains a license to practice, a right to practice. This right is not absolute or unqualified or natural; rather, it is subordinate to the police power of the state, which may control and regulate the practice of medicine in order to safeguard the public health and welfare. Health professionals may be disciplined by appropriate medical authorities, and have their licenses suspended or revoked in order to protect the public from incompetence, deception, or fraud. Reporting impaired physicians is important because the stakes for the public are so high. With professional rights of licensure come responsibilities to the public and to the profession.

Physician impairment is defined by the American Medical Association (AMA) (1973) as the inability to practice medicine with reasonable skill and safety because of physical or mental illness, including deterioration through the aging process, loss of motor skills, and the excessive use or abuse of drugs and alcohol.

Of these causes, chemical dependency has become the most frequently recognized reason for physician impairment; alcohol is the most commonly abused drug. It is unknown how many physicians abuse alcohol; however, it has been estimated that as many as 10% of all physicians have an alcohol problem (Simon, 1987, p. 432).

This chapter focuses on the impaired health professional, which includes the physician, but also other health professionals working in a general hospital. The impairments include primarily the abuse of alcohol or other drugs, mental or emotional illnesses, sexual offenses, gambling and other addictive behavior, and criminal behavior. Physical illness that impairs the health professional is not discussed. Mental or emotional illness may include organic mental disorder, psychosis, or a severe personality disorder that affects a health professional's ability to practice effectively within the hospital setting.

Organic mental illness or psychosis may clearly impair the professional; however, the physician may have a serious personality disorder, such as a passive-aggressive, antisocial, or borderline personality disorder, that is not so obvious, but that prevents the physician from working effectively and cooperatively with colleagues or from following the rules or guidelines of the hospital. The physician or health professional, because of such emotional disorder, may not get records in on time, attend staff meetings as required, or communicate effectively with colleagues in order to provide proper care of patients. This chapter is not concerned with those health-care professionals who do not keep up with the literature or newer treatment modalities, but do not have a mental or emotional impairment.

There are federal and state guidelines for reporting colleagues or peers who appear to be impaired (Health Care Quality Improvement Act, 1986). In Pennsylvania, for example, according to the Medical Practice Act of 1985, physicians have a statutory duty to report impaired colleagues or peers to the State Board of Medicine when there is "substantial evidence" of professional impairment (see also Moyer,

1987). If reported in good faith and without malice, immunity is granted from any resulting civil or criminal liability; in addition, failure to report such information can result in a fine.

Generally, physicians are reluctant to report apparently impaired colleagues. They appear to be concerned about liability for reporting, despite the promise of immunity in most jurisdictions. Three reasons for such physician reluctance to report colleagues may be as follows: (1) they fear identification with the professional or the procedure, fearing that others might subsequently report them as impaired (Walzer, 1990); (2) they fear being accused of "snitching" on colleagues as a "Big Brother" might do; and (3) they fear bringing economic ruin to a colleague and his or her family by such reporting, with its attendant consequences (Talbott, 1982).

The major ethical question to be addressed is the degree to which a health-care professional must be disturbed in order to be reported as impaired. What is the risk of harm to patients if the physician is not reported? What is the risk of harm to the health professional and his or her reputation and/or family if reported? The legal issue is the potential liability faced by those physicians or health-care professionals who report or who fail to report an impaired colleague. How should the reporting be done? Under what circumstances? And to whom? Some nonreporting health-care professionals not only may violate the ethical and professional standards of patient care, but also may violate criminal sanctions in some states, especially with respect to the sexual exploitation of patients. Thus an impaired health professional may pose ethical, legal, criminal, and licensing questions that need to be considered and discussed.

## NATURE OF THE IMPAIRMENT

Health professionals may be impaired as the result of a number of factors or causes. Impairment is defined as the loss of a function, where a person's ability to practice is diminished in value, strength, quality, or excellence. When the professional is impaired, the implication is that treatment may help to restore proper functioning. Impairment is to be distinguished from disability, which is defined as the inability to work, or, in law, as a legal incapacity.

Physicians and other health-care professionals with psychosis or serious mental disorders are readily recognized by peers, and they often come to official attention because of the severity of their mental disorders. Those impaired by substance abuse, particularly alcohol abuse, may be more difficult to identify until the abuse becomes excessive or extreme. Perhaps the most difficult to identify as impaired are those health professionals with personality disorders that appear subtly to affect performance. Some will become inappropriately involved with patients through sexual exploitation; others with passive-aggressive features will sabotage their own and others' efforts within the hospital by resisting change or through nonadherence to regulations and guidelines that are meant for all professionals to follow. Some with paranoid personalities or borderline features will have great difficulty in working with peers and with other colleagues within the hospital, thereby negatively affecting the treatment of patients.

By far, the most common impairment in health professionals is that of substance abuse, particularly the abuse of alcohol. Many states offer physician-impairment programs for treatment of the impaired professional. Most of these programs focus on the treatment of substance abuse, alcoholism, or other addictive diseases, such as compulsive gambling. Most states also have provisions for treatment of the psychotic professional. However, very few states offer programs for the more subtly impaired physician who denies any disorder and is resistant to treatment, discipline, or advice from others. Those in this group are the most difficult to identify and to manage within a physician-impairment program.

When a professional becomes involved in criminal behavior and is identified through arrest, the mechanisms for identification and reporting to proper agencies are clear. When a professional becomes involved in a malpractice action that reflects unethical behavior or "moral turpitude," such as sexual exploitation of patients, the identification and reporting mechanisms are also clear. A more difficult task may arise when the physician is suspected of abusing drugs or alcohol. Many substance abusers utilize denial as a defense mechanism and unless they are caught "red-handed" or exhibit a pattern of impaired judgment or behavior with respect to patients, they may be difficult to identify, and thus to be reported to the proper agencies or boards so that they might be disciplined or treated.

There are four major reasons for identifying the impaired physician and providing treatment for any health professional.

1. To promote the welfare of patients.
2. To save the lives and professional abilities of colleagues, and to restore these colleagues to good health.
3. To assure the competency and reliability of practitioners so that the art and science of the profession are maintained and enhanced.
4. To preserve the considerable investment society has made in the training of each professional (Steindler, 1987).

Most state medical societies devote most, if not all, of their attention to the treatment of chemical dependence, primarily alcoholism. Psychiatric problems are included only when they are associated with alcoholism or drug addiction. In an AMA survey in 1986, responses from 30 state society programs revealed that two thirds do handle some cases of major psychiatric disorders, such as depression; but it was clear that overall the concentration continued to be on substance abuse and dependence (Steindler, 1987). Some states have developed specific physician-impairment programs covering compulsive gambling, sexual exploitation of patients, and treatment of general psychiatric disorders without substance or alcohol abuse.

## REPORTING THE IMPAIRED PROFESSIONAL

Guidelines for reporting the impaired professional exist in federal and state legislation, as well as in codes and bylaws of professional organizations and associations. An example of state guidelines is the Pennsylvania Medical Practice Act of 1985, which provides, "Any hospital or health care facility, peer or colleague who has substantial evidence that a professional has an active disease for which the professional is not receiving treatment, is diverting a controlled substance or is mentally or physically incompetent to carry out the duties of his/her license, shall make or cause to be made a report to the Board" (sec. 422.2[f]).

A physician who is treating the impaired professional in an "approved treatment program" is exempt from the mandatory reporting requirements. The Pennsylvania law also provides that anyone who reports "in good faith and without malice" shall be immune from any civil or criminal liability arising from such a report (sec. 422.4[f]). State mandatory reporting laws generally provide such immunity for those who report, though some do not. State law also provides that anyone who fails to report within a reasonable time from receipt of knowledge of impairment shall be fined not more than $1000.

Federal guidelines exist through the Health Care Quality Improvement Act of 1986. This act sets out the requirements for reporting physicians whose professional competence is compromised and for sharing the information with licensing authorities and hospitals. There appear to be three basic needs for this federal legislation:

1. A need to improve the quality of medical care in view of the increasing occurrence of medical malpractice. This appears to be a national problem, and one that is greater than most states can handle by themselves.
2. A national need to restrict incompetent physicians from moving from state to state without making known their previous performance that had been detrimental to patients.
3. A need to give incentives and protection to physicians engaging in peer review, as they are currently discouraged by the threat of liability under federal antitrust law.

The federal legislation also protects the individuals who report professional impairment, as they are immune from damages and civil liability, unless the report is false and known to be false by the reporter (sec. 11111[a][2]). The federal law does not interfere with the state reporting laws, but expects the states to conform their standards to the federal guidelines for the sake of efficiency. States are also required to modify their statutes when preempted by the federal legislative guidelines. The advantage of federal legislation is that the states are now part of an improved network or national data bank that allows the screening of incompetent or impaired physicians who relocate to other jurisdictions, where their previous problems are unknown (Walzer, 1990).

Guidelines for reporting impaired colleagues are also established through professional associations and organizations. The American Psychiatric Association's (APA) *Principles of Medical Ethics, with Annotations Especially Applicable to Psychiatry* (1985a) state, "A physician shall deal honestly with patients and colleagues, and shall strive to expose those physicians deficient in character or competence, or who engage in fraud or deception" (sec. II, p. 2). The annotations also state, "Special consideration should be given to those psychiatrists who, because of mental illness, jeopardize the welfare of their patients and their own reputations and practices. It is ethical, even encouraged, for another psychiatrist to intercede in such situations" (p. 4). Further, the opinions of the APA Ethics Committee on the Principles of Medical Ethics (1985b) provide, "A physician should expose, without fear or favor, incompetent or corrupt, dishonest or unethical conduct on the part of members of the profession." Further, "One who believes a fellow psychiatrist is a potential danger to his patients should report this to the appropriate organizational component" (annot. 3).

The AMA's Model Impaired Physician Treatment Act of 1985 mandates the reporting of impaired physicians by the medical society only when the impairment constitutes a danger to the public. The AMA Council on Mental Health (1973) makes the following recommendations:

> It is the physician's ethical responsibility to take cognizance of a colleague's inability to practice medicine adequately by reason of physical or mental illness, including alcohol or drug dependence . . . When the physician is unable to make a rational assessment of his ability to function professionally, it becomes essentially the responsibility of his colleagues to make that assessment for him, and to advise him whether he should obtain treatment and curtail or suspend his practice.

The recommendations may be implemented in one of several ways:

1. By discussion of the problem with other physicians.
2. By referral of the problem to the medical staff of the hospital in which the affected physician serves.
3. By referral of the problem to a specific committee in the state or county medical society if the physician is not a member of the hospital staff.
4. By referral of the problem to the appropriate licensing body in the state if the physician is not a medical society member.

Thus, if the individual physician cannot be persuaded informally to seek help, and discussion of the problem with other physicians proves fruitless, the problem should be taken up by the medical staff of the hospital in which the affected physician serves. If that avenue is not feasible, or if the physician is not a member of a hospital staff, a specially designated committee of the state or county medical society should be consulted. If the medical society is unable or unwilling to act, or if the physician is not a medical society member, the matter should be referred to the appropriate licensing body in the state.

Despite these legal mandates and ethical considerations approved by the AMA and the APA, psychiatrists and other physicians are resistant to reporting, and often reluctant to report, colleagues who are involved in unethical conduct or whom they believe to be alcoholics, dependent on drugs, or emotionally or mentally disordered. They fear legal retaliation for exposing their colleagues. For example, civil liability may ensue for the tort of defamation when a statement is made concerning a physician that imputes a lack of the quality or skill that the public has a right to expect of people in this profession (Prosser, 1971). The interest at stake is the physician's reputation.

Physicians are generally given qualified immunity as a defense to such a charge of defamation. This means that they are not held liable for conduct that otherwise would be actionable because they are acting to further some interest of social importance that is entitled to protection, even at the expense of uncompensated harm to the physician's reputation. The only requirement is that the reporting be done in good faith and without malice. This means that the reporter's belief in the truth of what is reported, the purpose for saying it, and the manner of publication are all to be considered. The privilege is lost if the publication is not made primarily for the purpose of furthering the interest that is entitled to protection.

Physicians not only are professionally obligated, but also legally mandated, to report on their allegedly impaired colleagues. The law reflects a priority given to the interest in public health and welfare over the interest in a physician's reputation. Though the costs may be personal suffering and economic loss to the physician, they are outweighed by the benefits to the physician (treatment), to the patient (protection from harm), to the profession (retention of integrity), and to the public-at-large (information and protection). Most states have developed a virtual immunity for the reporting professional if the appropriate guidelines are followed, and, in fact, no physician reporters have been successfully sued (Simon, 1987).

In the final analysis, the real fear a physician or hospital should experience when considering reporting a possibly impaired colleague is not that of legal retaliation for reporting, but of negligence or civil liability for not reporting or for not taking some corrective action against the colleague who is posing, or should be known to pose, a risk to patient care.

According to federal guidelines, and almost all medical practice acts, a hospital has an express duty to report the impairment of a health-care professional. The hospital, as a corporation, has a duty to review periodically a physician's professional competence. Where the corporate entity breaches such duty and thereby proximately causes injury to a patient, the hospital may be held liable for damages to the patient if the impaired physician was not reported or was not kept from working directly with patients. The landmark case in this area is *Darling v. Charleston Community Memorial Hospital* (1965), in which the Supreme Court of Illinois held that a hospital has an independent corporate responsibility to carry out its bylaws to restrict the privileges of suspected impaired professionals. Under *Darling,* legal liability of the hospital staff is incurred if the staff did not restrict the privileges of a negligent physician and a patient subsequently was harmed.

## DISCIPLINING AND TREATING THE IMPAIRED PROFESSIONAL

Most states have developed, through their professional associations, treatment programs for impaired professionals. Physicians are encouraged to refer themselves when impairment occurs. However, for the resistant physician, referrals from colleagues, hospital administrators, insurance carriers, licensing boards, or family members are encouraged and accepted by the treatment facility for the impaired professional (Moyer, 1987).

In Pennsylvania, the Medical Practice Act of 1985 gives authority and responsibility to the Medical Board for disciplining physicians who are unable to practice medicine with reasonable skill and safety by reason of illness, drunkenness, or excessive use of drugs, narcotics, chemicals, or any type of material, or as a result of any mental or physical condition. The board is given similar responsibility for other health-care professionals regulated by the board. The board is also authorized to establish rules and regulations for the review and approval of medically directed, nonprofit, voluntary treatment programs for impaired physicians. The Medical Board's authority to discipline physicians and other professionals ranges from a private reprimand to revocation of license, plus appropriate fines. Included in this authority is the ability, by adjudication and order, to limit or otherwise restrict a license or to require the physician to submit to care, counseling, or treatment by a physician or physicians designed by the board (Steindler, 1987). The board may deny an application for a license if the applicant is the subject of a disciplinary proceeding.

The physician's license to practice may be limited or restricted by the board as follows:

1. The physician may practice only under the supervision of another specified physician.
2. The physician may not prescribe, dispense, or administer controlled substances.
3. The physician may not perform surgical procedures.
4. In some cases, especially that of a psychiatrist who has sexually exploited patients, the physician may not treat juveniles or members of the opposite sex.

The physician whose license has been suspended as the result of legal commitment because of mental incompetency or some type of impairment shall, at reasonable intervals, be afforded an opportunity to demonstrate to the board a capacity to resume a competent practice of medicine with reasonable skill and with safety to patients.

The AMA has developed model state legislation, the Model Impaired Physician Treatment Act, which provides for the funding of administrative expenses of the medical society's program, and mandates the reporting of names of impaired physicians by the society only when the impairment constitutes a danger to the public. The model bill clearly distinguishes impairment caused by alcoholism, drug abuse, or mental illness from professional incompetence, and it stipulates that physicians who participate in or have successfully completed treatment for their impairing illnesses shall not be excluded from membership on a hospital medical staff solely because of such treatment.

Other major provisions include the following:

1. Recognition by the regulatory board of the state medical society's program as the appropriate referral source for disposition of those cases that come to the board's attention and require therapeutic handling.
2. Periodic joint review by the board and the society's program administrators of impaired physicians' cases, with confidentiality of physicians' names assured.
3. Sharing of the society program's statistical information with the board and immunity for the medical society and its members for their actions in carrying out program functions.

It must be remembered that the purpose of physician-impairment laws includes the protection of society (specifically, the patient) and the encouragement of treatment of the impaired professional, rather than merely the punishment or disciplining of the suspected impaired professional.

A number of papers have been written describing the treatment and outcome of treatment of impaired physicians (Talbott, Gallegos, Wilson, & Porter, 1987; Arboleda-Florez, 1984; Arana, 1982). One study (Shore, 1982) involved a group of 34 impaired physicians on probation, and showed that treatment was effective for three fourths of those suffering from alcoholism, substance abuse, or major mental illness. The essential components of the treatment program included an attempt at rapid and early detection, a comprehensive medical and psychiatric evaluation, required ongoing treatment, and active, long-term follow-up by the Medical Board.

## GENERAL PHILOSOPHICAL AND ETHICAL CONSIDERATIONS

In addition to the legal aspects of reporting suspected impaired colleagues, there are ethical and moral issues to be discussed. When considering whether or not to report a colleague suspected of being impaired, the physician is often guided by both practical and theoretical considerations, and may also be guided by general ethical principles that include, but are not limited to, a "utilitarian" or "deontological" approach.

Under a utilitarian approach, an act is judged right or wrong based on the results the act brings about. The consequences of the action, and not the act itself, determine the morality of the act. According to John Stuart Mill (1861), one should act in such a way as to promote, as a result of the action, the greatest happiness for the greatest number affected by that action. This generalized benevolence subordinates the individual to the common good. Everyone is treated equally, and individuals are counted as measurable units. Happiness, the desired end, is defined as the promotion of pleasure and the prevention of pain. One calculates the consequences empirically, and without regard for a priori principles, since moral rules derive their status entirely from the fact that following them will generally maximize happiness.

One problem with this approach is that these empirical observations are often inaccurate and uncertain; for example, how to deal with the fact that what is pleasurable to one person may be painful to another, and how to predict a chain of events with calculated certainty. The utilitarian physician, however, when contemplating whether to report a possibly impaired colleague, would calculate and weigh the consequences of this action, and would conclude that an impaired physician should be reported, since more good consequences would follow from reporting than from not reporting.

The utilitarian physician might reason in any of the following ways. First, reporting would enable the impaired physician to obtain treatment, whereas not reporting would allow the impaired physician to go untreated. Second, reporting would ensure that patients would not be harmed before actions are taken to remove the impaired physician from practice, whereas not reporting would mean waiting for a patient to suffer damage that might have been avoided. Third, reporting would help the medical profession retain its integrity as a self-regulating association, whereas not reporting when harm results might call the effectiveness of that function into question. Fourth, reporting would satisfy the public-at-large, which wants (and needs) to be kept informed, whereas not reporting would outrage the public, which would feel deceived.

Under a deontological approach, an act is right or wrong because of the principle it embodies. It is the overriding principle of obligation or duty, and not the consequences of the act, that determines the morality of the act. According to Kant (1949/1785), an ethical duty should be consistent with the supreme moral principle, the categorical imperative—that one's act is such that everyone in similar circumstances should do the same thing on the same principle, as if the principle of one's act were to become a universal law of nature. Such a universal law should be followed without exception and without contradiction. A moral actor should treat others as ends in themselves and never as means; he or she would recognize the dignity of every individual.

One problem with this approach arises when there are two duties that conflict, one of which must be sacrificed in favor of the other. For example, one must opt between the duty to report an impaired colleague, which may result in humiliation of the colleague, and the duty to respect the colleague's professional reputation, which would entail shirking the duty to report. The deontological physician, however, contemplating whether or not to report a possibly impaired colleague, would reason according to principles, and would conclude that an impaired colleague should be reported since the duty to report is consistent with the supreme moral principle.

The deontological physician might reason in the following way. The question to ask is whether someone else in such a position should also report on the same principle, as if the imperative were a universal moral law. If protection of a physician's reputation means that an impaired physician's need for treatment is ignored, then the impaired physician is not shown respect, but is treated as a means to an end— the end being the protection of the non-reporter's own reputation, giving in to the fears of identification and/or retaliation. Because there is an exception to this duty to respect a professionals' reputation, it cannot be a universal moral law. On the other hand, there is no exception or contradiction to the duty to report. Thus all physicians should report their impaired colleagues.

Therefore, under either ethical theory, the philosophical physician would come to the same conclusion, albeit from different reasoning, that reporting the impaired physician is ethical and proper. Philosophically or theoretically, one can muse and talk about the morality of reporting, but practically speaking, physicians harbor a certain reluctance to report.

There seems to be a clash between the ethical principles adopted by the medical profession (the rules and laws that say one should report a colleague) and the real practices of the profession (the actual responses of physicians who do not wish to report). The final question is one of responsibility. Because the medical community has been given the privilege of being self-regulating, physicians must be guardians of their profession and of each other, if not of the patients they serve. Even though physicians are resistant to "snitch" laws and to reporting colleagues, according to the AMA statistics, colleagues in fact are the primary source of reports of physician impairment (AMA, 1973).

## THE ROLE OF THE FORENSIC PSYCHIATRIST

When a physician is suspected by colleagues, the hospital administration, or legal authorities of having an impairment that affects the ability to practice safely in the community, a forensic psychiatrist may be consulted to assess the mental state of the physician and his or her competency to practice medicine. A forensic psychiatrist may be called upon by the hospital administration when the hospital suspects that a physician is impaired as a result of mental illness, personality disorder, or substance abuse. A forensic psychiatrist also may be called by the physician or the physician's attorney to rebut a prior report that impairment exists. Finally, he or she may be called by the Medical Board or the licensing authority to provide an independent examination to help the board determine what actions to take against the suspected impaired physician.

Depending on the role assigned to the forensic psychiatrist, a number of procedural issues arise in conducting such an examination. First, the psychiatrist must identify his or her position to the physician being examined. The psychiatrist must indicate the source of referral and to whom a report will be sent. He or she must inform the physician that nothing that is said within the context of the examination can be held secret or confidential. All information gathered in the course of the examination will be subject to inclusion in a report that will be sent to the agency or the individual requesting the examination and evaluation.

The examining psychiatrist must also indicate that the possibility exists that the psychiatrist may testify in the course of a hearing regarding the competency of the physician to practice medicine.

A direct examination of the suspected impaired professional is necessary, but usually not sufficient, to conduct a thorough and comprehensive evaluation of the physician's competency to practice medicine. The examining psychiatrist should request appropriate records from the hospital, other physicians, psychiatrists, or treatment agencies in order to obtain a full and comprehensive assessment of the professional in question. He or she also may wish to interview significant members of the physician's family, as well as colleagues with whom the physician has worked. Some health professionals may be reluctant to discuss their observations and the opinions of their colleagues, but they should be strongly encouraged to provide as much information as possible in order that the suspected impaired professional can be assessed properly. Failure to conduct a thorough and comprehensive assessment may lead to erroneous conclusions that may negatively affect the colleague in question.

What liability does the forensic psychiatrist have in assessing a suspected impaired physician if the assessment is incomplete and the conclusions are inappropriate? If the assessment is negligently performed and the conclusions and recommendations improperly determined, and the physician is denied privileges or his or her reputation is negatively affected, the assessing psychiatrist may be subject to liability for negligent professional work that resulted in damage to the person assessed. No such lawsuits have yet been brought, but peer review of forensic assessments and forensic testimony is ongoing. It is likely that greater scrutiny will be paid to the manner in which forensic assessments are conducted and to whether standards of care are met by the assessing psychiatrist. Therefore, it is essential for any forensic psychiatrist involved in the evaluation of colleagues or peers who are suspected of being impaired to conduct a thorough and complete evaluation according to standards and guidelines accepted by other forensic psychiatrists.

Generally, such assessments are covered by the immunity clauses in state and federal laws affecting reporting of impaired professionals. However, the assessing psychiatrist is not the reporter in such cases. It is expected that the psychiatrist conducting such an assessment will adhere to generally accepted standards of care in order to avoid a negligent conclusion that might negatively affect a colleague with respect to impairment or competency.

## CASE EXAMPLES

### Case 1

A 48-year-old, married psychiatrist, father of four children, was accused of sexually exploiting a 33-year-old, single female teacher who had been his patient for five years. She complained to her attorney that for the past two years the psychiatrist had had regular sexual intercourse with her in his office at the hospital, following their weekly therapy sessions. She stated that she loved the physician and believed that he would leave his wife and family in order to marry her. When she realized that her wish was only a fantasy, she became depressed and suicidal. She required hospitalization, during which she told the attending psychiatrist about her extratherapeutic relationship with her former therapist. She also told her attorney that she wanted to sue her psychiatrist to keep him from exploiting other patients in a similar way.

The attorney consulted with the attending psychiatrist, and together they decided to approach the therapist. The attorney told the therapist that he would not pursue the matter in court if the doctor would agree to seek treatment in a special group of impaired physicians who had admitted to having sexual contact with their patients. The attorney also asked the therapist to pay his client a small sum of money to repair the emotional damage that was caused by the therapist's sexual involvement with her. The attending psychiatrist told the therapist that the patient was going to report the unethical behavior to the county medical society and to the APA, and that the patient also was planning to alert the licensing board about the behavior so that the board might mandate sanctions against the therapist.

The initial psychiatrist, wishing to avoid lengthy and painful litigation, agreed to make restitution to the patient and to submit himself for therapy in the impaired-physicians group. Reports were given to the medical society, to the APA, and to the licensing board. Because of the psychiatrist's willingness to admit his errant behavior and to obtain treatment in order to avoid similar behavior with other patients, he was given a mild sanction by the medical society and his license was not suspended; rather, his practice was restricted to adult male patients. At the conclusion of his two years of treatment, with the approval of the group therapist, and following a favorable report by an assessing forensic psychiatrist that he was safe to resume full practice of psychiatry, the restrictions on his license were removed.

This is an example of an ideal case in which lengthy, costly, and painful litigation is avoided when the impaired physician agrees readily to treatment and to help to restore the damage he caused to his former patient. In most cases, psychiatrists initially deny that they had any sexual contact with patients and begin a lengthy and difficult court battle, which often is lost or a settlement is negotiated following years of pretrial activities. Cooperative efforts, when an impaired physician exhibits unethical behavior, can be productive and helpful for all concerned.

**Case 2**

A 55-year-old physician began to drink excessively after his wife died following a lengthy illness. He was clearly depressed, but would not seek help from his colleagues at the hospital. He became increasingly irritable, short-tempered, and verbally abusive to patients. He began his hours later in the morning and began to leave early. His colleagues were concerned about his depression, but also about his increasingly difficult behavior. When he arrived at the hospital one day to consult in an emergency situation, he was noted to be in a clearly intoxicated state. The head nurse called a backup physician to take care of the emergency and to consult with the physician, who had become increasingly impaired in his ability to care for his patients. He was brought before the medical staff following a series of meetings to determine what should be done. It was decided to have a forensic psychiatric examination to determine the extent of the physician's illness and his increased alcohol intake, and he was given the option of being so examined or resigning from the medical staff. Because he believed, in his denial process, that nothing was wrong with him, he agreed to the examination. During the psychiatric assessment, the physician was initially antagonistic and resistant, but soon found relief in verbalizing his difficulties and expressing his grief over the loss of his wife. He then was able to recognize that he was depressed, and agreed to treatment.

He was placed on temporary suspension of hospital privileges until the treatment was complete.

This case illustrates a very common phenomenon in hospital medical practice. Physicians are human and can be subject to the same pressures of life and death as are their patients. Denial is a common mechanism of defense. However, a skillful forensic psychiatrist, recognizing the sensitivity of such an examination, usually allows several hours in which to work through the denial and to reach the painful core that cries out for help.

Other examples could illustrate the more difficult and problematic cases. Some physicians, with severe personality disorders, fight the accusations of their impairment for many years, frustrating the efforts of the hospital and the staff to deal effectively with them. Ultimately, the responsibility for the regulation of medical privileges for physicians working in general hospitals rests with the hospital administration, in order to protect the welfare of the patients and to preserve the integrity of the physicians.

## CONCLUSIONS AND RECOMMENDATIONS

It is ethical for a physician or health-care professional to report the impairment of a colleague when the impairment presents a substantial risk to the safety of patients or patient care. Early identification of the impaired physician is essential for proper treatment and the alleviation of symptoms.

It is essential for physicians to preserve the integrity of their profession and to protect the welfare of their patients. If a colleague poses a risk to either the profession or patient care, that colleague should be reported, disciplined, and treated, and restored to practice following successful treatment. The concern about immunity or liability for reporting is considerable, but may be reduced significantly through immunity laws and by following appropriate guidelines established by medical boards, state legislatures, and licensing authorities. Thus it is ethical, legal, and medically appropriate to report an impaired colleague in order to protect the welfare of the patients, preserve the integrity of the profession, and restore the colleague to professional competency.

## REFERENCES

American Medical Association, Council on Mental Health. (1973). The sick physician: Impairment by psychiatric disorders, including alcoholism and drug dependence. *JAMA, 223,* 684–687.

American Psychiatric Association. (1985a). *The principles of medical ethics, with annotations especially applicable to psychiatry.* Washington, DC: American Psychiatric Press.

American Psychiatric Association. (1985b). *Opinions of the ethics committee on the principles of medical ethics, with annotations especially applicable to psychiatry.* Washington, DC: American Psychiatric Press.

Arana, G. W. (1982). The impaired physician: A medical and social dilemma. *General Hospital Psychiatry, 4,* 147–154.

Arboleda-Florez, J. (1984). The mentally ill physician: The position of the Canadian Psychiatric Association. *Canadian Journal of Psychiatry, 29,* 55–59.

*Darling v. Charleston Community Memorial Hospital,* 33 Ill.2d 326, 211 N.E.2d 253 (1965), *cert. denied,* 383 U.S. 946 (1966).

Health Care Quality Improvement Act of 1986, 42 USCS, secs. 11101 *et seq.* (1989, plus Supp. 1991).

Kant, E. (1949). *Fundamental principles of the metaphysic of morals* (Trans.). Indianapolis, IN: Bobbs-Merrill. (Originally published 1785.)

Mill, J. S. (1861). *Utilitarianism.* London, England: Longman, Green.

Moyer, J. H. (1987). The Medical Practice Act of 1985. *Pennsylvania Medicine, 90,* 69–76.

Pennsylvania Medical Practice Act of 1985, 63 PA. Cons. Stat. Ann. sec. 422.4 (Purdon, 1989).

Prosser, W. (1971). *Law of torts.* St. Paul, MN: West.

Shore, J. H. (1982). The impaired physician: Four years after probation. *JAMA, 248,* 3127–3130.

Simon, R. I. (1987). *Clinical psychiatry and the law.* Washington, DC: American Psychiatric Press.

Steindler, E. (1987). Impaired health professionals: State of the art. *Maryland Medical Journal, 36,* 217.

Talbott, G. D. (1982). The impaired physician and intervention: A key to recovery. *Journal of the Florida Medical Association, 69,* 793.

Talbott, G. D., Gallegos, K. V., Wilson, P. O., & Porter, T. L. (1987). The Medical Association of Georgia's Impaired Physician Program: Review of the first one thousand physicians: Analysis of specialty. *JAMA, 257,* 2927–2930.

Walzer, R. (1990). Impaired physician: An overview and update of the legal issues. *Journal of Legal Medicine, 11,* 131–171.

# 14

## Child Abuse Reporting in the General Hospital

LINDA T. CAHILL,
LEAH E. HARRISON,
LYNN D. HAMBERG, AND
CAROL R. PERLMAN

Reports of child abuse in the United States in 1991 involved 2.7 million children, or 4.1% of the population under eighteen (National Child Abuse and Neglect Data System, 1993). Violence directed against children is not a new phenomenon. In fact, there is evidence to suggest that prior to 1800, the majority of the world's children were subject to abandonment, neglect, cruelty, and other abuses, including infanticide (DeMause, 1974; Tucker, 1974). Moreover, there is little evidence that early efforts to protect children from wanton abuse were motivated by humane and moral principles. For example, in ancient Greece and Rome, children were viewed as the property of the state and were to be protected as long as they enhanced the welfare of the state (Doxiadis, 1989). To that end, the writings of Aristotle supported the protection of healthy infants, but suggested that no cripple be reared (Aristotle, translation, 1951).

There were isolated attempts in more recent history to punish those who abused children, although no provisions existed to protect the victims. In a notable example from 13th-century England, it was decreed, "If one beats a child until it bleeds, then it will remember, but if one beats it to death, the law applies" (DeMause, 1974, p. 42). In the 18th century, religious orders took the initiative in establishing asylums for abandoned children, the first widespread practical expression of

269

humanitarian concern for children's welfare (Doxiadis, 1989). Even in modern times, although attitudes toward children have changed and their treatment has improved, as Farson (1974) notes, our society continues to discriminate against children.

## THE RIGHTS OF CHILDREN

It is generally acknowledged that their successful progression from infancy through childhood depends on the nurturing children receive from their adult caretakers. In healthy human development, the parent responds to the physical and psychological needs of the child. For example, feeding, bathing, soothing, and holding satisfy, in part, the needs of the infant. In addition, the parent assumes the much broader role of child advocate by safeguarding the child's rights within the environment, protecting him or her from harm, and by representing and guiding the child in the family and in the community.

Children's needs are provided for by adults intuitively, or by training or prior experience. Children's rights are those privileges and assurances guaranteed them by societal agreement, custom, or law. It is important to note that no one is guaranteed optimal, or even good-enough, treatment in our society. In the practical sense, children have the "right" to a life free of abuse only because of laws written to uphold their need to be protected from danger.

Additionally, in our society, most individuals have the right to make choices. In the period from infancy through adolescence, however, it might be dangerous to safeguard the right to choose. That is, during childhood, the relative importance to provide for children's needs overrides the need to assure their rights of privacy and autonomy.

The family is the basic social unit associated with the survival of children. Within the family structure, Anglo-American law protects parents (or guardians) from constraints on or intrusions into the functioning of the family, thereby assuring the right of guardians freely to conduct nurturing and advocacy functions and to exercise decision making, in privacy, on behalf of their children. However, if the guardian fails to provide for the needs of the child, it becomes a matter of public concern. In that case, the state may take over in order to guarantee the child's rights (Solnit, 1982).

## CHILD ABUSE LEGISLATION; HISTORICAL PERSPECTIVE

It is only in the past 40 years in this country that concerns over the duty of the state to protect children and the power of state agencies to intervene in family life have become a matter of practical consideration and application. Removal of a child from a parent's custody because of flagrant battering was first authorized by a New York court in 1874, and then only because of a statute protecting animals from cruelty (Lazoritz, 1990).

Outside of the home, children's needs for protection were more apparent and readily recognized. For example, fair labor legislation prohibited children from working in hazardous industries, and limited the number of hours those under 16 years of age were allowed to work. However, such laws did not spark widespread public interest and concern for many decades. It took a medical report by Kempe, Silverman, Steele, Droegemueller, and Silver (1962) to achieve this. As a result of that publication, child physical abuse has become increasingly acknowledged as associated with other family problems, including child neglect, child sexual abuse, and failure to provide adequate nurturing, education, medical attention, and other supports for a child's growth.

The recognition among professionals and in the lay press of the problem of child abuse coincided with the civil rights movement of the 1960s. During that period, a widely held belief developed that state and national governments had a responsibility to protect the disadvantaged; children whose families could not provide for them fell into this group. In the years following, it was recognized among professionals that people who abused children only rarely were cruel and sadistic. These abusive parents often had been abused themselves, and were burdened by severe psychological and family problems. In effect, child abuse was deemed a symptom of systemic and family dysfunction. It was reasoned that if appropriate rehabilitative and supportive services were established to assist troubled families, parents might be more effective in protecting and nurturing their children (Steele & Pollock, 1974).

A U.S. Senate Subcommittee on Children and Youth was created in 1971 that concluded that there was a need for a coherent federal role in the identification, prevention, and treatment of abused and neglected children. The work of the subcommittee resulted in the signing of the Child Abuse Prevention and Treatment Act of 1974. In the original Senate bill, "abuse" and "neglect" intentionally were left undefined, as the law was intended to support clinical services and research, and not to be regulatory or punitive. The House version, however, included a definition involving physical and mental injury. But even then, there was no illusion that all families meeting the definition that focused on physical abuse would receive help from the limited funding available (Hoffman, 1979). Notably, when it came time for the states to define "child abuse" in order to qualify for federal funds, the U.S. Department of Health, Education, and Welfare required that it be defined even more broadly, and, in addition, mandated reporting by a long list of professionals.

In 1975, an expert commission that studied child abuse reporting expressed concern that the broadened definition and mandatory reporting scheme would result in a flow of reports to the child welfare agencies that would overwhelm the system (Newberger, 1983; Sussman & Cohen, 1975). In fact, the prevalence of child abuse is far greater than was anticipated in 1974, and the increase in reports has far exceeded these predictions. In 1967, approximately 7000 reports of child abuse and neglect were received nationwide. By 1978, reports had increased 100-fold. Even more sobering were estimates derived from household surveys of severe injuries inflicted on children ranging from one to four million incidents per year (Gelles, 1978). The pressure on professionals mandated to report suspected abuse and neglect has placed an extraordinary burden on child welfare agencies. These agencies investigate each case, and make recommendations for appropriate services based on their findings and, at their discretion, those of teachers, counselors, physicians, and other professionals involved with the child's care. In cases where the risk of injury is deemed significant, state-designated child welfare agencies can take the child into protective custody and recommend temporary placement.

## DEFINITIONS

Child "abuse" and "neglect" are defined in New York State by the New York Social Services Law [1983 & Supp. 1992, sec. 412(1)] and by the

New York Family Court Act [1983 & Supp. 1992, sec. 1012(1-3,f)]. An "abused" child is defined as a child less than 18 years of age whose parent or guardian "inflicts or allows to be inflicted upon such child physical injury by other than accidental means which causes or creates a substantial risk of death, or serious or protracted disfigurement . . . [or] commits, or allows to be committed, a sex offense against such child as defined in the penal law . . . ." A "neglected" child is one whose "physical, mental or emotional condition has been impaired or is in imminent danger of becoming impaired as a result of the failure of his parent [or guardian] to exercise a minimum degree of care." The parent or guardian must supply minimally adequate food, clothing, shelter, and education, and must provide for medical and dental care. The parent or guardian must not inflict excessive corporal punishment. The guardian may not misuse drugs so as to lose control of his or her actions, resulting in neglect or maltreatment of the child.

Significantly, "guardian" or "custodian" includes any person continually or at regular intervals found in the same household as the child. The social services law also identifies operators of day-care centers and other authorized agencies as persons legally responsible. "Mandated reporters" are those who, in their professional capacity, are likely to encounter situations in which abuse of children is identified or suspected. In such cases, mandated reporters by law must report suspicion of child abuse to the child protective agency. When the report is made in good faith, the mandated reporter has immunity from liability in most states. The New York Social Services Law (1983 & Supp. 1989, sec. 413) identifies a mandated reporter as follows: "Any physician, surgeon, medical examiner, coroner, dentist, dental hygienist, osteopath, optometrist, chiropractor, podiatrist, resident, intern, registered nurse, hospital personnel engaged in administration, examination, care or treatment of persons, a Christian Science practitioner, school official, social services worker, day care center worker, mental health professional, peace officer, police officer or law enforcement official, and psychologist."

Included in state child abuse laws is the reporting requirement for "suspicion" of abuse. That is, the mandated reporter is required to file a report when he or she has reason to believe that abuse may have occurred. This particular aspect of the reporting laws leaves little discretion for alternative interventions. Failing to report child abuse may result in civil liability based on a theory of professional malpractice that the child sustained further injury as a direct result of the professional's negligent failure to diagnose, treat, or act to mitigate the abuse. Notably, the violation of the statutory duty to report results in an irrebuttable presumption of negligence.

Criminal liability may also result from failure to report child abuse. The most common state-imposed penalty for failure to report is a jail sentence of six months or a $500 fine or both. Notably, however, in Maryland, failure to report child abuse is considered a felony, and carries a penitentiary sentence of 15 years.

## SUSPICION OF ABUSE

Consider the case of infant J., the youngest of seven children. At the age of three weeks, he was admitted to the pediatric ward with a fracture of the left humerus. His mother informed doctors that a right humerus fracture was identified when the baby was 10 days old. Consultation with specialists suggested that J. might have a metabolic bone disorder that could make him particularly prone to long-bone fractures with relatively minor trauma. The highly specialized tests are not available locally or quickly, nor are they guaranteed to identify the problem even if it exists. None of the older, verbal children reported abuse within the household, nor was there any evidence that they were victims of abuse.

There is no question but that two traumatic episodes were responsible for this child's injuries. Whether the trauma was related to intent to "punish" the infant or resulted from excessive use of force by an unsupervised child may never be known. Regular follow-up in a pediatric clinic would suffice to identify and treat any subsequent medical problem and to provide routine health care. In addition, suspicion of abuse requires a report to the state child-abuse registry. The child welfare agency has the power to investigate and to enforce compliance with recommended interventions, thereby assuring medical follow-up. There is no allowance under the law for the other option, which is not to report, nor would that necessarily be desirable. The child protective agency that investigated this case supported the medical recommendations. In addition, it recommended temporary placement of infant J. in foster care and a parenting-skills program for his mother and father. The agency noted correctly that there was considerable uncertainty about the nature of the events that resulted in the injury. Even if the infant had a bone disorder, everyone noted that excessive force on two separate occasions resulted in the long-bone fractures, and since both events were unwitnessed, the injuries might indeed have been inflicted with intent to harm.

In contrast, consider the case of a mother who was waiting for medical care in a busy pediatric emergency room with her sick, crying three-year-old child. She was observed hitting him and screaming at him several times. The child was eventually diagnosed as having a severe ear infection, which undoubtedly resulted in significant pain and caused him to be irritable and behaviorally unmanageable in a crowded emergency-room waiting area. After interviewing his tearful, overwhelmed mother, the child protection team social worker was able to provide immediate support and, at a subsequent visit, connected the family with vocational counseling and other indicated services.

In this case, professional discretion resulted in an alternative to reporting the case to the local child-abuse hotline. The family complied with recommendations, thereby avoiding being reported on a subsequent date to the child welfare agency. This plan is not without risk, however. If the family lived in substandard housing, if a parent abused drugs or alcohol to an extent sufficient to place the children in jeopardy, or if this child or other children in the household were often left unsupervised, such information would not be available without investigations that only the child welfare agency is authorized to carry out.

## EXACERBATING THE ABUSE

Melissa, nearly three years old, had an abnormal vaginal examination and repeatedly said "Papa touched me" when interviewed about possible abuse. After she was placed in foster care, she became withdrawn, and was often inconsolable. Her father and mother separated, and her father, who denied any abusive touching of his daughter, became increasingly despondent. He attended recommended therapy sessions, but was discharged from care because he denied responsibility for the abuse and the need for ongoing services. Unable to convince his wife and the court that he was innocent, he took his own life, saying in a final note that he could not live with the shame of the accusations despite the fact that they were false.

This is a tragic example of exacerbation of abuse. Several systems failed, perhaps unavoidably, to recognize the degree of pain endured by this family. The child protection agency focused on the welfare of the child, given the information at hand. The counseling agency saw no need to keep the child's father in therapy for abusing her since he adamantly denied guilt. In this case, well-intentioned decisions of several agencies resulted in irreversible disaster.

Although Weisberg and Wald (1986) have noted that abused or neglected children would be placed at significant risk without outside intervention, others have argued that such intervention often perpetuates the abuse. If a two-year-old child has been sexually abused and there is no identified perpetrator, the child protective agency, acting on behalf of the state, might justifiably choose to separate the child from the nuclear family, pending the results of lengthy investigations. Separation of a very young child from his or her mother at such a critical, early stage of development may arguably be a form of "abuse" to the child, this time the result of the actions of an imperfect, state-imposed child-advocacy system.

The mother or other family member may not actually be responsible for the abuse, but parent and child are separated for lack of existing viable alternatives, while the state intrudes upon the privacy of the family and makes recommendations for rehabilitative services. The ultimate goal is to reunite the family. Although attempts are made by the state to help provide the family with parenting programs, homemaking services, vocational training, substance abuse counseling, psychiatric services, and legal services, as indicated, these services are far too scarce to meet the demand. Moreover, individuals within a family must be willing to accept such services, and may do so only in the interest of cooperating with the system in order that their children can return home. The family or any of its members may not perceive the need for these services and will not benefit from them. Young mothers may themselves be the products of dysfunctional families.

They are confused and angered by the events following the identification of abuse of their children. Services for these parents who have been separated from their children must be able to deal with the negative feelings generated by the separation and must provide them with the coping resources they previously lacked.

## ASSESSMENT OF RISK OF ABUSE AND NEGLECT

There are four stages in working with children at risk of abuse and neglect: identification, evaluation, immediate protection, and long-term planning. Certain well-described behavioral indicators may flag children who are being abused or who are at risk. Children may be reluctant to go home, may run away repeatedly, may be aggressive or withdrawn, or may manifest low self-esteem. Such nonspecific indicators of family dysfunction should alert those who observe them to investigate further in order to determine if abuse or neglect is a possible cause. The medical and teaching professions are the first-line observers of child abuse and neglect. Teachers have access to children for six hours a day, nine months a year, and can observe subtle signs, such as a change in behavior or school performance, sleeping in class, depression, or repeated signs of physical injury. Medical providers have an opportunity to observe and interpret the nature of injuries in children, depression, behavioral problems, failure to thrive, evidence of neglect (poor hygiene, improper clothing), and lack of adequate medical care.

There apparently is no legal protection for mandated reporters, nor are families required to submit to in-depth investigation, in a case where so-called "predictors" of child abuse are present. Families can be urged to take their children for medical evaluation if these predictors are identified, but they cannot be made to do so. If families fail repeatedly to follow through on recommendations, then they may be seen as "neglecting" their children. Because these families can escape follow-up by the system that identified them by disconnecting their telephones, changing their addresses and their source of health care, or intentionally giving false identifying information, the professional must act quickly and expeditiously in reporting cases when suspicion of abuse exists.

There are other "red flags" that may predict child neglect, such as substance abuse by the parent(s). In these families, the parent's time and resources are devoted to drug-seeking activities, and not the care of the children. However, the professional who suspects but has no direct knowledge of such drug-abusing activity in the family cannot in good faith make a report of the risk of child abuse unless the child manifests concrete evidence of dysfunction.

Abused children may attempt suicide or abuse alcohol or drugs. Sexually abused children may demonstrate sophisticated or unusual sexual behavior or knowledge. Neglected children may be hungry or tired all the time, have improper clothing, and be dirty and unkempt. At the time of a physical examination, physically abused children may have characteristic injuries in the shape of the abusing instrument or an explanation for an injury that is inconsistent with the findings. Sexually abused children may have characteristic tears, scars, or other evidence of abusive contact in the rectogenital area. More serious sequelae of abuse include pregnancy and sexually transmitted diseases, such as gonorrhea, syphilis, chlamydia, hepatitis, and the acquired immunodeficiency syndrome (AIDS). The risk of death to young victims of sexual abuse is increasing as the incidence of infection by the human immunodeficiency virus (HIV) among perpetrators increases. Evaluation can be complicated by the lack of findings, along with unconvincing histories in young victims. In approximately 70% of the cases of child sexual abuse where there is a clear history, there will be no medical evidence of injury (Muram, 1989).

## EVALUATION

Evaluation should include an interview and physical examination appropriate to the age and development of the child. Evidence gathering is far more clear-cut in cases of physical abuse where bruises and fractures are readily identified than in the area of sexual abuse. Most providers of medical services are hesitant to examine children for evidence of sexual abuse, either for lack of experience, or because of a reluctance to provide expert witness testimony in court. Children may undergo multiple examinations, by providers with varying degrees of expertise, in order to "confirm" suspicion.

In the course of evaluating an abused child, it is essential to determine the risk for further abuse before discharging the child to his or her home. Such investigations and resultant conclusions are fraught with pitfalls, not only in the case of preverbal or nonverbal children who are unable to relate abusive events or to name perpetrators, but in many other instances as well.

A 12-year-old child, accompanied by her mother, presents to the emergency room with fever and pharyngitis. In the course of her examination, doctors determine that she is 20 weeks pregnant. The child says that she thought she was pregnant and that she wants to keep the baby. Upon learning of her oldest daughter's pregnancy, her 26-year-old mother asserts, "I can't be watching her all the time. She is out on the streets and she doesn't listen." The child firmly denies that she was forced into sexual acts, stating that she has been sexually active since the age of 10 and that she does not know who fathered the baby. Her mother is very clear about her willingness to support her daughter's decision to live at home after the baby is born and to assist her with child care.

The law in most states would support an allegation of lack of supervision and maternal neglect in the case of a 10-year-old child who is sexually active while in her mother's care. The family court might rule that the child be placed in foster care, as the child's mother has no interest in counseling or family therapy.

In this case, the law requires that the case be reported to the child welfare agency for lack of supervision. In considering available options, a decision to keep this family together is desirable and justified. Irrespective of the allegations (and ultimately the findings) against the mother, short- and long-term plans must be set into motion for this family by the child welfare agency on the order of the family court. The short-term goals might include enrolling the 12-year-old in prenatal care and child-care classes and monitoring her attendance in school. Counseling for the mother-to-be should include goal setting and long-term vocational guidance so that she can start to plan for her own future and that of her child. Because her mother might be guilty of neglect, the siblings of the 12-year-old must be evaluated for evidence of abuse or neglect. This family will need careful follow-up and intervention as indicated.

## CULTURAL DIFFERENCES

The starved, tattered, or bruised child presents the classic picture of neglect or abuse regardless of nationality, race, or ethnic origin. Most cases of child maltreatment are less obvious, however, and identification must include an appreciation of the cultural context of the act of omission or commission. There is no universal standard for appropriate child care, or even for child abuse and neglect. This gives rise to a dilemma. If cultural differences are ignored, then one risks assuming that only one or two sets of cultural standards of discipline of children constitute the norm, and that all others are, at the very least, unacceptable, and at the very worst, abusive. On the other hand, forgiving inhumane treatment of children in the name of cultural differences could result in a lesser standard of care for some children (Korbin, 1987).

John, 11 years of age, stayed out until 2:00 A.M. one morning. When he arrived home, his frantic parents beat him with a belt about the trunk and legs, leaving him covered with red and blue welts. During a routine examination the following day, the doctor questioned his mother about the bruises. She was a caseworker for the local field office of the child protective agency charged with investigating allegations of abuse and neglect. The violence of the disciplinary measures she and her husband used was, in her opinion, justified by her child's reckless disobedience. She said that she was disciplined with physical force (as was everyone she knew) in the country of her birth, and that she had "turned out all right."

Intrafamily violence is an accepted way of life in too many families. In the case above, alternative forms of discipline might be employed that would not result in physical injury, and might even have more impact on changing behavior. Reeducation is needed to alter the pattern of physically abusive behavior toward children so that the next generation of parents will learn to practice nonabusive, alternative forms of discipline and will not jeopardize the lives of their own children.

## PITFALLS OF CHILD ABUSE LEGISLATION

Child abuse legislation has been the subject of increasing controversy. Some critics believe the laws to be vague or imprecise, and that they result in overreporting (Goldstein, Freud, & Solnit, 1979). Newberger (1983) has observed that the system designed to handle only a fraction of the 60,000 reported cases per year in 1974 can never hope to address the millions of cases reported annually since the 1980s. Heymann (1986) has noted that the law does not allow those professionals who are mandated to report the option of exercising professional judgment about the appropriateness or implications of reporting. It is not even clear that interventions, particularly family disruptions, will have more positive than negative effects, even in cases where families are "bad."

In another study, which looked at the compliance of hospital personnel with the child abuse reporting laws, Newberger (1983) noted that underreporting was particularly prevalent in white, affluent families where the mother was the alleged perpetrator. He noted also that fewer than half of appropriate cases were reported; race and social class of the abuser were found to be more predictive of reporting than was the severity of the abuse. And in yet another study, Rabb (1981) found that physicians, nurses, and social workers were willing to report less severe examples of child abuse when they were presented with vignettes of lower-class families. It might be argued that the more affluent are subject to meeting a lesser standard of care. While the reasons are not totally clear, the continued underreporting of abuse in more affluent families has been explained, in part, by their greater success in masking abusive situations. In addition, wealthier families have less contact than do the poor with the social and other public agencies that might identify child abuse as they intervene on behalf of the latter families in other situations.

Katz, Ambrosino, McGrath, and Sawitsky (1977) defined several problems in the legal sphere. Since the child abuse laws are state laws, there are 51 sets of laws and judicial interpretations. Moreover, the definitions of child abuse and child neglect can vary, not only from state to state, but even among the jurisdictions of a single state. The provisions of the "neglect" laws are often imprecise and vague, and they cannot be operationalized to the minimum level of parental care tolerable. In some instances, the reporter becomes an accuser, a hazardous situation in states in which, in the above language, abuse is also part of the criminal code.

## FETAL ABUSE

In the past several decades, there has been a shift in emphasis from the rights and privileges of the mother to those of her unborn child. Historically, the paramount aim of obstetrics was the preservation of maternal health (see Rosenthal, 1992). However, recently the focus has shifted to the fetus as a second patient (Pritchard, MacDonald, Gant, & Williams, 1985).

Our increasing concerns over fetal rights are due, in part, to advances in technology that enable us to see the fetus, learn its sex, diagnose conditions that may require intrauterine surgery, and then perform that surgery (Nelson & Milliken, 1988). In addition, the medical profession has gathered substantial information about the effects of smoking, legal and illicit drugs, alcohol, diet, and environmental toxins on the developing fetus. The government becomes interested in the fetus after the period of viability (*Roe v. Wade,* 1973), about 24 weeks into gestation, when the fetus has the potential to live outside the uterus.

Separating the rights of the mother and her unborn baby is fraught with difficulties. Maternal–fetal conflicts can arise when the mother refuses physician-recommended treatments, does not seek prenatal care, or refuses to change behaviors, such as alcohol or drug abuse, that can be harmful to her unborn baby. The following case (Rosenthal, 1992) illustrates the difficulties inherent in applying statistical certainties to any individual case.

A woman with complete placenta previa (the placenta covering the outlet of the uterus) refused a cesarean section and blood transfusion despite the physician's predictions that without these interventions, she and her unborn child had a 50% and 99% risk, respectively, of dying. The court ordered that the unborn child have legal protection and that the mother undergo all procedures that physicians deemed necessary. She refused on religious grounds, disappeared from the hospital, and did well after giving birth, vaginally, to a healthy baby.

This case illustrates the inability of the medical profession to predict, with certainty, the outcome of high-risk pregnancy. On the other hand, the overwhelming probability that harm would come to both the baby and the mother resulted in physician recommendations of presumed lifesaving surgery.

There is ample precedent for court intervention in cases where religious beliefs endanger the life or welfare of a child. In those cases, in most states, the court takes custody of the child and orders the recommended interventions. On the other hand, in the case in which the child at risk is yet to be born, there are strong ethical arguments against forced procedures (Mahowald, 1989): (1) under the doctrine of informed consent, competent patients can accept or refuse procedures based on their understanding, (2) procedures such as cesarean section and blood transfusion carry their own risks, (3) individuals generally cannot be forced to have an invasive procedure to save someone else, (4) patients (mothers) have a right to their own bodily integrity, (5) the question as to whether the fetus is a "person" has not been settled in law.

The issues surrounding the conflicts between the rights of the mother and those of her unborn child are coming under increasing scrutiny as pressure mounts to reverse *Roe v. Wade* and to criminalize fetal abuse (Note, *Harvard Law Review,* 1988). In some states, the civil court will order custody of a pregnant woman (as in the case above) to optimize care to her unborn child (Rosenthal, 1992). However, in most states, including New York, the child abuse laws apply only to children from birth to 18 years of age. Action apparently may be taken only to protect the newborn who is considered endangered because of high-risk maternal behaviors during pregnancy.

## CONCLUSION

The past century has seen dramatic changes in the way that people treat children. Children are no longer viewed as little adults, but are recognized as helpless and vulnerable and as having special needs. Even more striking has been the increasing role of government in assuring that children grow up free of abuse by those charged with their care. But the system is not perfect, because, except in the most egregious cases of maltreatment, children can be subject to repeated exposure to abuse by laws that were designed both to protect them and to preserve the family unit.

No one claims to know what is "best" for children. What is known, however, is that the ability of a child to adjust to and overcome some of the immediate emotionally damaging effects of battering or sexual abuse is profoundly affected by the response of adults to those events. Interventions called for by the child protection laws include, for example, the use of supportive counseling to help guardians work through their own problems so they can be available to the child both practically and emotionally. In addition, long-term planning is built into the laws to allow guardians who were separated from their abused children to develop coping skills and other resources to care for and protect those children in the future. In this context, child abuse reporting laws must be viewed as offering new hope to hundreds of thousands of young people in this country who otherwise were surely doomed.

## REFERENCES

Aristotle. (1951). *The politics* (Book VII) (T. A. Sinclair, trans.). Harmondsworth, England: Penguin.

Child Abuse Prevention and Treatment Act of 1974, 42 U.S.C.A. secs. 5101 *et seq.*

DeMause, L. I. (1974). The evolution of childhood. In L. I. DeMause (Ed.), *The history of childhood.* New York: Psychohistory Press.

Doxiadis, S. A. (1989). Children, society and ethics. *Child Abuse and Neglect, 13,* 11–17.

Farson, R. (1974). *Birthrights.* New York: Macmillan.

Gelles, R. J. (1978). Violence toward children in the United States. *American Journal of Orthopsychiatry, 48,* 580–592.

Goldstein, J., Freud, A., & Solnit, A. (1979). *Before the best interests of the child.* New York: Free Press.

Heymann, G. (1986). Mandated child abuse reporting and the confidentiality privilege. In L. Everstine & D. Everstine (Eds.), *Psychotherapy and the law.* Orlando, FL: Grune & Stratton.

Hoffman, E. (1979). Policy and politics: The Child Abuse Prevention and Treatment Act. In R. Bourne & E. H. Newberger (Eds.), *Critical perspectives on child abuse.* Lexington, MA: Heath.

Katz, S. N., Ambrosino, L., McGrath, M., & Sawitsky, K. (1977). Legal research on child abuse and neglect: Past and future. *Family Law Quarterly, 11,* 151–184.

Kempe, C. H., Silverman, F. N., Steele, B. F., Droegemueller, W., & Silver, H. K. (1962). The battered child syndrome. *JAMA, 181,* 17–24.

Korbin, J. E. (1987). Child abuse and neglect: The cultural context. In R. F. Helfer & R. S. Kempe (Eds.), *The battered child.* Chicago, IL: University of Chicago Press.

Lazoritz, S. (1990). Whatever happened to Mary Ellen? *Child Abuse and Neglect, 14,* 143–149.

Mahowald, M. (1989). Beyond abortion: Refusal of Caesarian section. *Bioethics, 3,* 106–121.

Muram, D. (1989). Child sexual abuse: Relationship between sexual acts and genital findings. *Child Abuse and Neglect, 13,* 211–216.

National Child Abuse and Neglect Data System, Working Paper 2, 1991 Summary Data Component. (1993). National Center on Child Abuse and Neglect, Washington, D.C.

Nelson, L., & Milliken, N. (1988). Compelled medical treatment of pregnant women. *JAMA, 259,* 1060–1066.

Newberger, E. H. (1983). The helping hand strikes again: Unintended consequences of child abuse reporting. *Journal of Clinical Child Psychology, 12,* 307–311.

Note (1988). Developments in the law. *Harvard Law Review, 101,* 994–1012.

New York Family Court Law sec. 1012 (McKinney 1983 & Supp. 1992).

New York Social Services Law secs. 412–413 (McKinney 1983 & Supp. 1992).

Pritchard, J. A., MacDonald, P. C., & Gant, N. F. (1985). *Obstetrics.* Norwalk, CT: Appleton-Century-Crofts.

Rabb, J. (1981). Reporting child maltreatment: The context of decision making among physicians, social workers, teachers and nurses. *Dissertations Abstracts International, 42,* 7-A, 3306.

*Roe v. Wade,* 410 U.S. 113 (1973).

Rosenthal, M. B. (1992). Maternal-fetal conflicts: A modern dilemma. In D. H. Schetky & E. P. Benedek (Eds.), *Clinical handbook of child psychiatry and the law.* Baltimore, MD: Williams & Wilkins.

Solnit, A. J. (1982). Children, parents and the state. *American Journal of Orthopsychiatry, 52,* 496–505.

Steele, B. F., & Pollock, C. B. (1974). A psychiatric study of parents who abuse infants and small children. In R. E. Helfer & C. H. Kempe (Eds.), *The battered child.* Chicago, IL: University of Chicago Press.

Sussman, A., & Cohen, S. J. (1975). *Reporting child abuse and neglect: Guidelines for legislation.* Cambridge, MA: Ballinger.

Tucker, M. J. (1974). The child as beginning and end. In L. I. DeMause (Ed.), *The history of childhood.* New York: Psychohistory Press.

Weisberg, R., & Wald, M. (1986). Confidentiality laws and state efforts to protect abused or neglected children: The need for statutory reform. In L. Everstine & D. Everstine (Eds.), *Psychotherapy and the law.* Orlando, FL: Grune & Stratton.

# 15

---

# Legal and Ethical Issues in Psychiatric Research

## CHRISTINA CASALS-ARIET

This chapter touches upon certain issues pertaining to psychiatric research in the general hospital. It is intended to give a brief overview of topics with which clinicians interested in carrying out research in the general hospital should be familiar. These include a brief summary of the history of regulations pertaining to research and investigative subjects, informed consent, competency, institutional review boards (IRBs), coercion in the research setting, and some of the decision-making steps that a person considering research must take.

Significant realization of ethical issues in medical research first came to widespread public attention at the Nuremberg trials of Nazi physicians in 1946. The Nuremberg Code comprised an early articulation of ethical standards to be followed in pursuing research. The three central requirements of the Nuremberg Code were that: (1) the voluntary consent of the person on whom the experiment is to be performed must be obtained; (2) the danger of each experiment must have been investigated previously by means of animal experimentation; and (3) the experiment must be performed under proper medical protection and management. It was required that research subjects have legal capacity to give consent, be free of undue influence, and possess sufficient knowledge to enable an understanding decision (see Appelbaum & Roth, 1982). These later came to be incorporated as elements of the doctrine of informed consent.

National codes that were developed subsequent to the Nuremberg Code contained many similarities, but also had enough deviations for it to become clear by the early 1960s that an international code was needed. Also, a flaw in the Nuremberg Code was the lack of a provision enabling research on patients without the legal capacity to consent. Thus, in 1964, the Declaration of Helsinki, adopted by the World Medical Association, answered the need for an international formulation of ethical standards (see generally Appelbaum & Roth, 1982). The declaration made a distinction between clinical research combined with professional care and nontherapeutic research. The 1964 code also allowed third-party consent to serve as a substitute for the consent of an incapacitated person.

For a time, such nonbinding codes remained the primary instruments addressing issues of research, consent, and competency. Few cases came before the courts, and such case law as did develop (e.g., *Kaimowitz v. Michigan State Department of Mental Health,* 1952) did not serve to resolve the issues.

What developed more substantially than case law were administrative regulations. A variety of events led to hearings and study groups within the Food and Drug Administration (FDA) and the National Institutes of Health (NIH), and in 1966 the NIH devised a uniform policy on the regulation of experimentation. The Public Health Service (PHS) (the parent body of the NIH) issued a statement requiring grant applicants to provide prior approval of any project submitted by a principal investigator (PI) or program director. This review would assure an independent determination of (1) the rights and welfare of the individual or individuals involved, (2) the appropriateness of the methods used to secure informed consent, and (3) the risks and potential benefits of the investigation.

This PHS statement became the benchmark for all regulations that followed. Various revisions were made over the years, but essentially from then on the requirement for research funded by the then Department of Health, Education, and Welfare, currently the Department of Health and Human Services (DHHS), was for a "decentralized, institution-based, prospective review of research, with informed consent explicitly required as part of the process of subject recruitment" (45 CFR sec. 46.101).

Regulations have grown in complexity. They now encompass such issues as details about review committees' makeup and reach, records, the manner of obtaining informed consent from subjects, and substituted consent.

## INFORMED CONSENT

Of the variety of issues addressed by the regulations, informed consent is of paramount importance; indeed, it is the foundation of any ethical research. A major principle underlying informed consent is autonomy. This principle promotes a number of benefits: protection of patients and subjects, avoidance of fraud and duress, encouragement of self-scrutiny by medical professionals, promotion of rational decisions, and involvement of the public (Appelbaum, Lidz, & Meisel, 1987).

From ethical roots, informed consent grew to be a legal doctrine as case law developed. The details are beyond the scope of this chapter, but suffice it to say that consent is more than merely the patient's agreement to research. There are two other essential features, namely, understanding and voluntariness. The patient must be given information in such a fashion that he or she can understand it, and must be situated in life such that his or her decision is freely made. These are complex notions.

To assist those involved in the early decision-making and planning stages of research, and to assist IRBs, the DHHS regulations specify what must be disclosed to subjects:

1. A statement that the study constitutes research, and an explanation of its purposes.
2. A description of risks and discomforts that are reasonably foreseeable.
3. A description of possible benefits to the subjects and to others.
4. A disclosure of appropriate alternative treatments, if any.
5. A statement describing the extent of confidentiality of records generated.
6. An explanation of whether compensation or treatment will be available if injuries occur.
7. A note as to whom to contact with questions or reports of injuries.
8. A statement clearly indicating the voluntary nature of participation and the subject's right to withdraw at any time.

With regard to the issue of voluntariness, the regulations require that consent be sought only under circumstances that provide the prospective subject (or the subject's legally authorized representative) sufficient opportunity to consider whether or not to participate, and that minimize the possibility of coercion or undue influence (see Appelbaum et al., 1987, p. 226). This does not afford much in the way of practical guidance. Similarly, the DHHS regulations require that information be given in language that subjects are likely to understand, though the specifics of how to accomplish this are not addressed. With reference to competency, the regulations provide that if patients are incompetent, their legally authorized representatives may consent on their behalf to research participation. The FDA regulations are essentially similar to these.

## COMPETENCY

As stated by Appelbaum and Roth (1982, p. 951): "The issue of competency to consent to therapeutic and experimental procedures has recently been propelled into the forefront of debate about medical and experimental ethics . . . however, the issue of competence . . . to consent to research is of relatively recent derivation and awaits generally acceptable attempts at definition." The authors proceed to explain the four commonly used standards for competency: (1) evidencing a choice, (2) factual understanding of the issues, (3) rational manipulation of information, and (4) appreciation of the nature of the situation.

These four standards of competency are arranged in hierarchic fashion according to a continuum of strictness. The least rigorous standard is evidencing a choice. By this criterion, the subject need only indicate a willingness to participate in the study. The next standard is a subject's factual understanding of the issues, which requires that the subject have the cognitive ability to comprehend the nature of the procedure, attendant risks, available options, that there is a choice to make, and the consequences of participation or nonparticipation.

The third standard is the rational manipulation of information, one step more rigorous in the hierarchy. By this criterion, how the subject uses information in the decision-making process is evaluated. Finally, the strictest standard is the appreciation of the nature of the situation; that the subject appreciate the consequences of giving or withholding consent, have a sense of who he or she is and why he or she is agreeing, recognize in a mature fashion the implications of alternative courses of action, and appreciate both cognitively and affectively the nature of the thing to be decided.

The real decision to be made by a potential researcher with regard to competency is which standard to use. The decision is one of policy: Which values are of paramount importance to a particular group? Among these are autonomy, rational decision making, beneficence, respect for persons, justice, encouragement of research, subject satisfaction, and ease of administration. The potential researcher needs to spend time thinking about these issues before making the decision to proceed.

## INSTITUTIONAL REVIEW BOARDS

In addition to considering the important questions of informed consent and competency, potential researchers must anticipate and plan for the process of submitting papers to and appearing before a hospital's IRB. The 1981 revisions of the DHHS regulations require that IRBs have at least five members with varying backgrounds, in order to promote complete and adequate review of research activities. Members must be demographically varied, and some must be knowledgeable about applicable case law and regulations, as well as standards of professional conduct. At least one member must not be on the staff of the institution.

The role of the IRB is to review proposed projects to ensure conformity with federal regulations. Of note are the following criteria: minimization of risk to subjects; reasonable relationship between existing risks and anticipated benefits; equitable selection of subjects; appropriately requested and documented informed consent; monitoring subject privacy and safety, if needed; and protection of vulnerable subjects from undue coercion.

## ADDITIONAL CONCERNS

Even when the hurdles of consent and IRB approval are surmounted, other problems exist for the researcher. Of great significance, and involving difficult and delicate decisions, are the fine lines between research and therapeutic functions and between encouragement and coercion. Each challenges the researcher to develop communication skills that allow open and full exchanges with potential subjects.

The boundary between research and therapy can be blurred. Investigators may feel discomfitted by putting patients in research projects that may not allow physicians to care fully for their patients (Appelbaum et al., 1987, pp. 244–245). Equally problematic for researchers is the type of interaction with patients required in these situations: open talks about unsure outcomes. Physicians are usually not taught the skills needed to engage in this type of discussion. Psychiatrists may have an advantage in this regard, although that is by no means a certainty.

A concern of a different kind than nondisclosure is that of coercion. The nature of the physician–patient relationship, especially as it has been historically, is one of inequality. Patients are vulnerable to the knowledge and "power" of the doctor, and thus are frequently dominated by the will of doctors regarding medical decisions.

This difficulty is conceivably intensified in patients who are research subjects. They may be exceptionally ill and thus feel even more helpless in the face of their disease and the doctor's enhanced, "healing" stature. It is the researcher's responsibility to monitor the potential for coercion and to guard against it. In circumstances in which the researcher is recruiting possible subjects for a project with which he or she is intimately involved, the physician may not be the person who should give information and obtain informed consent. Because the danger of self-interest is potentially too great to allow the physician the degree of disinterest needed to make a balanced presentation, someone else should talk with the prospective subjects. Even if the investigator is able to achieve a balanced approach, the possibility of an appearance of impropriety still necessitates a disinterested person's involvement with the process of consent.

## CASE EXAMPLES

The following case vignettes will serve to highlight some of the issues discussed.

## Case 1: Deteriorating Cognitive Impairment

Mrs. C.B. is a 70-year-old, married mother of three and grandmother of four. She was admitted to the medical–psychiatric unit of the hospital for further evaluation and workup of her declining mental state. Mrs. B.'s family has been aware for more than a year that her memory and ability to function have been steadily declining. She has begun to wander out of the house without proper clothing, and generally to be inattentive to personal care. Lately her condition has worsened and the family can no longer manage her.

Physical examination and laboratory testing were unrevealing. After an electrocardiogram and computed-tomography scan, as well as a period of observation, the diagnosis arrived at was Alzheimer's Disease. The medical–psychiatric unit of the hospital is testing a new, experimental drug for patients with early Alzheimer's disease, and the research team would like to try the medication on Mrs. B. What questions need to be considered in the decision-making process?

A primary issue presented in this situation, as in all cases of research, is that of informed consent. A necessary component of informed consent is competency, and Mrs. B.'s mental status is clouded to the point that her ability to give informed consent is impaired. She might be able to pass the least rigorous standard, evidencing a choice, but would that be sufficient to enter her into a research trial? Given her apparent inability to *understand* the relevant information, and to withstand even minor *duress or influence,* this standard would be insufficient.

Could the family be substituted as decision maker for Mrs. B.? What considerations would enter the balance? Have the family and Mrs. B. discussed treatment in the event of decline? Do they know how she felt before her dementia began? Has she signed a health-care proxy or living will? And what of risk–benefit considerations regarding the medication? Is Mrs. B. at great risk from receiving no treatment? Does the medication have few side effects, or pernicious ones? Is the medication known to be at all helpful, or with no appreciable effect to date? These are just a few of the factors that researchers, patients, and families must address. It is a complex process, one often of shades and gradations rather than clear answers.

In this case, assume that Mrs. B. has reliably expressed the view that she wants to be helpful to science, and that she trusts her children to know what is best. In addition, assume that although the benefit of the drug is currently questionable at best, the known side effects are minimal, and thus the risk is not great. Under such circumstances, substituted consent would be warranted.

## Case 2: Intermittent Psychosis

Mr. V.L. is a 38-year-old, single, unemployed, undomiciled man who was brought into the emergency room by the ambulance service. He had been found wandering the streets, shouting, muttering, and walking unheedingly into traffic. Upon examination, he was found to be grossly psychotic, delusional, and hallucinating. Convinced that he was the Invincible Man, he was certain that no harm could befall him and that ordinarily dangerous events were of no threat to him. Physical examination was unremarkable, and he was admitted to the inpatient psychiatric unit.

Mr. L. is well known to the hospital staff. He has a 20-year history of 22 prior hospitalizations, beginning when he was 18 years old. His pattern has been relatively consistent, and the nature of his illness, chronic undifferentiated schizophrenia, has not changed much. He becomes delusional and confused, is admitted to the hospital and treated with medication, and then improves. His thought processes stabilize, and he is discharged. Eventually, he stops coming to the follow-up clinic, he fails to take his medication, and his mental status declines. Although he is intelligent, when psychotic, he is incapable of rational decision making.

The members of the psychiatric staff are conducting research on a new potent antipsychotic medication. It is extremely effective in relapsing, noncompliant patients like Mr. L., and they are anxious to try him on the medication. What issues are involved in the decision-making process?

Again, informed consent is an important issue. Can Mr. L. give informed consent, or does his current psychotic state render him incompetent? At his most florid moments, Mr. L. is incompetent, unable to make a rational choice. Can a substitute decision maker be appointed? Here, history is helpful. The staff knows that with a period of conventional medication, Mr. L. will improve rather rapidly. His thought processes will clear. Also, although at risk when on the street, he is not a threat to himself or others while in the hospital, and thus there is no emergent need to treat him with a research drug. When he improves, he can be approached regarding a trial of the medication. Finally, although the new medication is extremely effective, assume it carries a significant risk of a certain potentially serious side effect. In this instance, the research team should wait until Mr. L. improves. The team members may then speak with him and arrive at a mutually satisfactory plan, in which he would receive a trial of medication, with assurances that side effects will be closely monitored and treated immediately.

The question to consider would have been different had the patient not been known, for then his pattern of response would be unclear. Also, had the patient been a more imminent risk, relentlessly bent on self-destruction and unresponsive to conventional medication, the risk–benefit analysis would perhaps shift in favor of a trial of the new medication.

In both of the cases, an additional issue for consideration is that of coercion. In the case of Mrs. B., the possibility exists that coercion would become a factor were there no family or an unconcerned family. Physicians must always safeguard their patients, and potential research subjects, from overzealousness on the investigators' part, whether or not the patient is able to do so for himself or herself. With Mr. L., coercion might be a factor when he is psychotic, but as he improves, he can become a participant in the decision making. Waiting, in this case, will make a difference, whereas with Mrs. B., waiting will not, as Mrs. B. will not improve.

These cases serve to delineate a few of the questions that arise in research. It is axiomatic that prudence and thoughtfulness in the decision-making process are of utmost importance.

## SUMMARY

The topics discussed are just some of the issues presented in the process of research in the general psychiatric setting. The list is not exhaustive, and more remains to be said about these topics. Nonetheless, the foregoing may provide a point of departure for psychiatrists in their thinking when they need to make decisions about research.

Researchers need to be aware that such decision making entails several steps, each an integral part of the entire process of conducting an investigation. First, of course, is whether or not to embark on the project at all. The questions of primary concern in this regard are whether the information to be gained will be of substantial merit, and whether the benefits to be gained outweigh the potential risks. Also to be considered is the likelihood that the project will receive IRB approval.

The next tier of decision making involves outlining the specific project. Clearly, the more complex and intricate the proposed study, the more time consuming and costly it will be. Also, the higher the risk involved, the more difficulty there will be with IRB approval, and perhaps with getting subjects.

Once these decisions have been made, there still remain the many subsequent decisions about individual patients. This involves constant vigilance and awareness of the need for caution. Each person must be approached as an individual, with a fresh, unbiased explanation. With every encounter, the physician must consider again the issues of informed consent, risk, possible benefits, and potential harm.

All in all, research is a demanding occupation, requiring thought on many levels. Yet there is no better way to advance our knowledge, so vital for the continued care of the many patients whose illnesses require understanding and treatment.

## REFERENCES

Appelbaum, P. S., Lidz, C. W., & Meisel, A. (1987). *Informed consent: Legal theory and clinical practice.* New York: Oxford University Press.

Appelbaum, P. S., & Roth, L. H. (1982). Competency to consent to research: A psychiatric overview. *Archives of General Psychiatry, 39,* 951–958.

Public Health Service, Department of Health and Human Services, Policy for Protection of Human Research Subjects, 45 C.F.R. §§ 46.101 *et seq.*

*Kaimowitz v. Michigan Dept. of Mental Health,* no. 73-19434-AW. Mich. Cir. Ct., Wayne Co. July 10, 1973, 1 MDLR Rptr. 147 (1976).

# Author Index

# Subject Index

304